PEDIATRICS, CHILD AND ADOLESCENT HEALTH

CHILDREN AND YOUTH

POST-TRAUMATIC STRESS DISORDER AND MOTOR VEHICLE CRASHES

PEDIATRICS, CHILD AND ADOLESCENT HEALTH

JOAV MERRICK - SERIES EDITOR
NATIONAL INSTITUTE OF CHILD HEALTH AND HUMAN DEVELOPMENT, MINISTRY OF SOCIAL AFFAIRS, JERUSALEM

Child and Adolescent Health Yearbook 2012
Joav Merrick (Editor)
2012. ISBN: 978-1-61942-788-4 (Hardcover)
2012. ISBN: 978-1-61942-789-1 (e-book)

Child Health and Human Development Yearbook 2011
Joav Merrick (Editor)
2012. ISBN: 978-1-61942-969-7 (Hardcover)
2012. ISBN: 978-1-61942-970-3 (e-book)

Child and Adolescent Health Yearbook 2011
Joav Merrick (Editor)
2012. ISBN: 978-1-61942-782-2 (Hardcover)
2012. ISBN: 978-1-61942-783-9 (e-book)

Tropical Pediatrics: A Public Health Concern of International Proportions
Richard R Roach, Donald E Greydanus, Dilip R Patel, Douglas N Homnick and Joav Merrick (Editors)
2012. ISBN: 978-1-61942-831-7 (Hardcover)
2012. ISBN: 978-1-61942-840-9 (e-book)

Child Health and Human Development Yearbook 2012
Joav Merrick (Editor)
2012. ISBN: 978-1-61942-978-9 (Hardcover)
2012. ISBN: 978-1-61942-979-6 (e-book)

Developmental Issues in Chinese Adolescents
Daniel TL Shek, Rachel CF Sun and Joav Merrick (Editors)
2012. ISBN: 978-1-62081-262-4 (Hardcover)
2012. ISBN: 978-1-62081-270-9 (e-book)

Positive Youth Development: Theory, Research and Application
Daniel TL Shek, Rachel CF Sun and Joav Merrick (Editors)
2012. ISBN: 978-1-62081-305-8 (Hardcover)
2012. ISBN: 978-1-62081-347-8 (e-book)

Understanding Autism Spectrum Disorder: Current Research Aspects
Ditza A Zachor and Joav Merrick (Editors)
2012. ISBN: 978-1-62081-353-9 (Hardcover)
2012. ISBN: 978-1-62081-390-4 (e-book)

Positive Youth Development: A New School Curriculum to Tackle Adolescent Developmental Issues
Hing Keung Ma, Daniel TL Shek and Joav Merrick (Editors)
2012. ISBN: 978-1-62081-384-3 (Hardcover)
2012. ISBN: 978-1-62081-385-0 (e-book)

Transition from Pediatric to Adult Medical Care
David Wood, John G Reiss, Maria E Ferris, Linda R Edwards and Joav Merrick (Editors)
2012. ISBN: 978-1-62081-409-3 (Hardcover)
2012. ISBN: 978-1-62081-412-3 (e-book)

Adolescence and Behavior Issues in a Chinese Context
Daniel TL Shek, Rachel CF Sun, and Joav Merrick (Editors)
2013. ISBN: 978-1-62618-614-9 (Hardcover)
2013. ISBN: 978-1-62618-692-7 (e-book)

Advances in Preterm Infant Research
Jing Sun, Nicholas Buys and Joav Merrick
2013. ISBN: 978-1-62618-696-5 (Hardcover)
2013. ISBN: 978-1-62618-775-7 (e-book)

Child Health and Human Development: Social, Economic and Environmental Factors
Leslie Rubin and Joav Merrick (Editors)
2013. ISBN: 978-1-62948-166-1 (Hardcover)
2013. ISBN: 978-1-62948-169-2 (e-book)

Children, Violence and Bullying: International Perspectives
Joav Merrick, Isack Kandel and Hatim A Omar (Editors)
2013. ISBN: 978-1-62948-342-9 (Hardcover)
2013. ISBN: 978-1-62948-345-0 (e-book)

Chinese Adolescent Development: Economic Disadvantages, Parents and Intrapersonal Development
Daniel TL Shek, Rachel CF Sun and Joav Merrick (Editors)
2013. ISBN: 978-1-62618-622-4 (Hardcover)
2013. ISBN: 978-1-62618-694-1 (e-book)

Chronic Disease and Disability in Childhood
Joav Merrick
2013. ISBN: 978-1-62808-865-6 (Hardcover)
2013. ISBN: 978-1-62808-868-7 (e-book)

Environmental Health Disparities in Children: Asthma, Obesity and Food
Leslie Rubin and Joav Merrick (Editors)
2013. ISBN: 978-1-62948-122-7 (Hardcover)
2013. ISBN: 978-1-62948-135-7 (e-book)

Environmental Health: Home, School and Community
Leslie Rubin and Joav Merrick (Editors)
2013. ISBN: 978-1-62948-155-5 (Hardcover)
2013. ISBN: 978-1-62948-158-6 (e-book)

Guidelines for the Healthy Integration of the Ill Child in the Educational System: Experience from Israel
Yosefa Isenberg
2013. ISBN: 978-1-62808-350-7 (Hardcover)
2013. ISBN: 978-1-62808-353-8 (e-book)

Internet Addiction: A Public Health Concern in Adolescence
Artemis Tsitsika, Mari Janikian, Donald E Greydanus, Hatim A Omar and Joav Merrick (Editors)
2013. ISBN: 978-1-62618-925-6 (Hardcover)
2013. ISBN: 978-1-62618-959-1 (e-book)

Playing with Fire: Children, Adolescents and Firesetting
Hatim A. Omar, Carrie Howell Bowling and Joav Merrick (Editors)
2013. ISBN: 978-1-62948-471-6 (softcover)
2013. ISBN: 978-1-62948-474-7 (e-book)

Promotion of Holistic Development of Young People in Hong Kong
Daniel TL Shek, Tak Yan Lee and Joav Merrick (Editors)
2013. ISBN: 978-1-62808-019-3 (Hardcover)
2013. ISBN: 978-1-62808-040-7 (e-book)

University and College Students: Health and Development Issues for the Leaders of Tomorrow
Daniel TL Shek, Rachel CF and Joav Merrick (Editors)
2013. ISBN: 978-1-62618-586-9 (Hardcover)
2013. ISBN: 978-1-62618-612-5 (e-book)

Break the Cycle of Environmental Health Disparities: Maternal and Child Health Aspects
Leslie Rubin and Joav Merrick (Editors)
2013. ISBN: 978-1-62948-107-4 (Hardcover)
2013. ISBN: 978-1-62948-133-3 (e-book)

Human Developmental Research: Experience from Research in Hong Kong
Daniel TL Shek, Cecilia Ma, Yu Lu and Joav Merrick (Editors)
2014. ISBN: 978-1-62808-166-4 (Hardcover)
2013. ISBN: 978-1-62808-167-1 (e-book)

School, Adolescence and Health Issues
Joav Merrick, Ariel Tenenbaum and Hatim A. Omar (Editors)
2014. ISBN: 978-1-62948-702-1 (Hardcover)
2014. ISBN: 978-1-62948-707-6 (e-book)

Adolescence and Sexuality: International Perspectives
Joav Merrick, Ariel Tenenbaum and Hatim A. Omar (Editors)
2014. ISBN: 978-1-62948-711-3 (Hardcover)
2014. ISBN: 978-1-62948-724-3 (e-book)

Child and Adolescent Health Yearbook 2013
Joav Merrick (Editor)
2014. ISBN: 978-1-63117-658-6 (Hardcover)
2014. ISBN: 978-1-63117-668-5 (e-book)

Adoption: The Search for a New Parenthood
Gary Diamond and Eva Arbel (Israel)
2014. ISBN: 978-1-63117-710-1 (Hardcover)
2014. ISBN: 978-1-63117-713-2 (e-book)

Adolescence: Places and Spaces
Myra F. Taylor, Julie Ann Pooley and Joav Merrick (Editors)
2014. ISBN: 978-1-63117-847-4 (Hardcover)
2014. ISBN: 978-1-63117-850-4 (e-book)

Pain Management Yearbook 2013
Joav Merrick (Editor)
2014. ISBN: 978-1-63117-944-0 (Hardcover)
2014. ISBN: 978-1-63117-959-4 (e-book)

Child Health and Human Development Yearbook 2013
Joav Merrick (Editor)
2014. ISBN: 978-1-63117-939-6 (Hardcover)
2013. ISBN: 978-1-63117-958-7 (e-book)

Born into this World: Health Issues
Donald E. Greydanus, Arthur N. Feinberg, and Joav Merrick (Editors)
2014. ISBN: 978-1-63321-667-9 (Hardcover)
2014. ISBN: 978-1-63321-669-3 (e-book)

Caring for the Newborn: A Comprehensive Guide for the Clinician
Donald E. Greydanus, Arthur N. Feinberg and Joav Merrick (Editors)
2014. ISBN: 978-1-63321-760-7 (Hardcover)
2014. ISBN: 978-1-63321-781-2 (e-book)

Environment and Hope: Improving Health, Reducing AIDS and Promoting Food Security in the World
Leslie Rubin and Joav Merrick (Editors)
2014. ISBN: 978-1-63321-772-0 (Hardcover)
2014. ISBN: 978-1-63321-782-9 (e-book)

Pediatric and Adolescent Dermatology: Some Current Issues
Donald E Greydanus, Arthur N Feinberg and Joav Merrick (Editors)
2014. ISBN: 978-1-63321-853-6 (Hardcover)
2014. ISBN: 978-1-63321-863-5 (e-book)

A Pediatric Resident Pocket Guide: Making the Most of Morning Reports
Arthur N. Feinberg
2015. ISBN: 978-1-63482-141-4 (Softcover)
2015. ISBN: 978-1-63482-186-5 (e-book)

Tropical Pediatrics: A Public Health Concern of International Proportions Second Edition
Richard R. Roach, Donald E. Greydanus, Dilip R. Patel and Joav Merrick (Editors)
2015. ISBN: 978-1-63463-381-9 (Hardcover)
2015. ISBN: 978-1-63463-404-5 (e-book)

Child and Adolescent Health Issues (A Tribute to the Pediatrician Donald E Greydanus)
Joav Merrick (Editor)
2015. ISBN: 978-1-63463-574-5 (Hardcover)
2015. ISBN: 978-1-63463-576-9 (e-book)

Child and Adolescent Health Yearbook 2014
Joav Merrick, MD (Editor)
2015. ISBN: 978-1-63482-162-9 (Hardcover)
2015. ISBN: 978-1-63482-206-0 (e-book)

Child Health and Human Development Yearbook 2014
Joav Merrick (Editor)
2015. ISBN: 978-1-63482-163-6 (Hardcover)
2015. ISBN: 978-1-63482-207-7 (e-book)

Behavioral Pediatrics, 4th Edition
Donald E. Greydanus, Dilip R. Patel, Helen D. Pratt, Joseph L. Calles Jr., Ahsan Nazeer and Joav Merrick (Editors)
2015. ISBN: 978-1-63483-027-0 (Hardcover)
2015. ISBN: 978-1-63483-052-2 (e-book)

Disability, Chronic Disease and Human Development
Joav Merrick
2015. ISBN: 978-1-63483-029-4 (Hardcover)
2015. ISBN: 978-1-63483-057-7 (e-book)

Caribbean Adolescents: Some Public Health Concerns
Cecilia Hegamin-Younge and Joav Merrick (Editors)
2015. ISBN: 978-1-63483-341-7 (Hardcover)
2015. ISBN: 978-1-63483-343-1 (e-book)

Adolescence and Health: Some International Perspectives
Joav Merrick (Editor)
2015. ISBN: 978-1-63483-791-0 (Hardcover)
2015. ISBN: 978-1-63483-808-5 (e-book)

Youth Suicide Prevention: Everybody's Business
Hatim A. Omar (Editor)
2015. ISBN: 978-1-63483-786-6 (Softcover)
2015. ISBN: 978-1-63483-820-7 (e-book)

Chronic Disease and Disability: The Pediatric Kidney
Donald E Greydanus, Vimal Master Sankar Raj, Joav Merrick (Editors)
2016. ISBN: 978-1-63483-793-4 (Hardcover)
2015. ISBN: 978-1-63483-809-2 (e-book)

Child and Adolescent Health Yearbook 2015
Joav Merrick (Editor)
2016. ISBN: 978-1-63484-512-0 (Hardcover)
2016. ISBN: 978-1-63484-543-4 (e-book)

Child Health and Human Development Yearbook 2015
Joav Merrick (Editor)
2016. ISBN: 978-1-63484-513-7 (Hardcover)
2016. ISBN: 978-1-63484-544-1 (e-book)

Pain Management Yearbook 2015
Joav Merrick (Editor)
2016. ISBN: 978-1-63484-515-1 (Hardcover)
2016. ISBN: 978-1-63484-545-8 (e-book)

Children and Childhood: Some International Aspects
Joav Merrick (Editor)
2016. ISBN: 978-1-63484-587-8 (Hardcover)
2016. ISBN: 978-1-63484-594-6 (e-book)

Children and Adolescents: Future Challenges
Daniel TL Shek, Tak Yan Lee, and Joav Merrick (Editors)
2016. ISBN: 978-1-63484-616-5 (Hardcover)
2016. ISBN: 978-1-63484-627-1 (e-book)

Adolescence: Positive Youth Development Programs in Chinese Communities
Daniel TL Shek, Florence KY Wu, Janet TY Leung, and Joav Merrick (Editors)
2016. ISBN: 978-1-63484-044-6 (Hardcover)
2016. ISBN: 978-1-63484-677-6 (e-book)

Sexuality: Some International Aspects
Joav Merrick and Donald E Greydanus (Editors)
2016. ISBN: 978-1-63484-707-0 (Hardcover)
2016. ISBN: 978-1-63484-719-3 (e-book)

Growing Up in the Middle East: The Daily Lives and Well-Being of Israeli and Palestinian Youth
Yossi Harel-Fisch, Ziad Abdeen and Miriam Navot
2016. ISBN: 978-1-63484-746-9 (Hardcover)
2016. ISBN: 978-1-63484-765-0 (e-book)

Chronic Disease and Disability: The Pediatric Heart
Donald E. Greydanus, Devika Malhotra and Joav Merrick (Editors)
2016. ISBN: 978-1-63484-828-2 (Hardcover)
2016. ISBN: 978-1-63484-842-8 (e-book)

Chronic Disease and Disability: The Pediatric Pancreas
Donald E. Greydanus, Manmohan K Kamboj and Joav Merrick (Editors)
2016. ISBN: 978-1-53610-055-6 (Hardcover)
2016. ISBN: 978-1-53610-065-5 (e-book)

Diabetes Mellitus: Childhood and Adolescence
Manmohan K Kamboj, Donald E Greydanus and Joav Merrick (Editors)
2016. ISBN: 978-1-53610-095-2 (Hardcover)
2016. ISBN: 978-1-53610-104-1 (e-book)

Chronic Disease and Disability: Abuse and Neglect in Childhood and Adolescence
Donald E Greydanus, Vincent J. Palusci and Joav Merrick (Editors)
2016. ISBN: 978-1-53610-129-4 (Hardcover)
2016. ISBN: 978-1-53610-142-3 (e-book)

Clinical Aspects of Psychopharmacology in Childhood and Adolescence, Second Edition
Donald E. Greydanus, Joseph L. Calles, Jr., Dilip R. Patel, Ahsan Nazeer, and Joav Merrick (Editors)
2016. ISBN: 978-1-53610-241-3 (Hardcover)
2016. ISBN: 978-1-53610-253-6 (e-book)

Child and Adolescent Health Yearbook 2016
Joav Merrick (Editor)
2017. ISBN: 978-1-53610-948-1 (Hardcover)
2017. ISBN: 978-1-53610-957-3 (e-book)

PEDIATRICS, CHILD AND ADOLESCENT HEALTH

CHILDREN AND YOUTH

POST-TRAUMATIC STRESS DISORDER AND MOTOR VEHICLE CRASHES

DONALD E. GREYDANUS,
ROGER W. APPLE,
KATHRYN WHITE
AND JOAV MERRICK
EDITORS

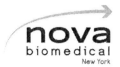

Copyright © 2017 by Nova Science Publishers, Inc.

All rights reserved. No part of this book may be reproduced, stored in a retrieval system or transmitted in any form or by any means: electronic, electrostatic, magnetic, tape, mechanical photocopying, recording or otherwise without the written permission of the Publisher.

We have partnered with Copyright Clearance Center to make it easy for you to obtain permissions to reuse content from this publication. Simply navigate to this publication's page on Nova's website and locate the "Get Permission" button below the title description. This button is linked directly to the title's permission page on copyright.com. Alternatively, you can visit copyright.com and search by title, ISBN, or ISSN.

For further questions about using the service on copyright.com, please contact:
Copyright Clearance Center
Phone: +1-(978) 750-8400   Fax: +1-(978) 750-4470   E-mail: info@copyright.com

NOTICE TO THE READER

The Publisher has taken reasonable care in the preparation of this book, but makes no expressed or implied warranty of any kind and assumes no responsibility for any errors or omissions. No liability is assumed for incidental or consequential damages in connection with or arising out of information contained in this book. The Publisher shall not be liable for any special, consequential, or exemplary damages resulting, in whole or in part, from the readers' use of, or reliance upon, this material. Any parts of this book based on government reports are so indicated and copyright is claimed for those parts to the extent applicable to compilations of such works.

Independent verification should be sought for any data, advice or recommendations contained in this book. In addition, no responsibility is assumed by the publisher for any injury and/or damage to persons or property arising from any methods, products, instructions, ideas or otherwise contained in this publication.

This publication is designed to provide accurate and authoritative information with regard to the subject matter covered herein. It is sold with the clear understanding that the Publisher is not engaged in rendering legal or any other professional services. If legal or any other expert assistance is required, the services of a competent person should be sought. FROM A DECLARATION OF PARTICIPANTS JOINTLY ADOPTED BY A COMMITTEE OF THE AMERICAN BAR ASSOCIATION AND A COMMITTEE OF PUBLISHERS.

Additional color graphics may be available in the e-book version of this book.

Library of Congress Cataloging-in-Publication Data

ISBN: 978-1-53611-102-6

Published by Nova Science Publishers, Inc. † New York

Contents

Dedication		xiii
Preface		xv
Introduction		1
Chapter 1	Introduction to post-traumatic stress disorder and motor vehicle crashes in children and adolescents: A historically delayed realization *Donald E Greydanus and Joav Merrick*	3
Section one: The killing fields		23
Chapter 2	The killing fields on the roads: Can we protect the teen driver? *Donald E Greydanus*	25
Chapter 3	Demographics *Kathryn White*	77
Chapter 4	Assessment of posttraumatic stress disorder in children and adolescents subsequent to motor vehicle crash *Kathryn White*	91
Chapter 5	Differential diagnosis and comorbid conditions *Adam J Mrdjenovich*	107
Chapter 6	The psychological impact of motor vehicle crashes (MVC) on children and adolescents *Roger W Apple*	119

Chapter 7	Assessment, early intervention and evidence-based treatments for posttraumatic stress disorder in children following motor vehicle accidents *Jennifer Kuhn, McKenna Corlis and Amy Damashek*	135
Chapter 8	Youth motor-vehicle collision survivors in the classroom *A Benton Darling*	153
Chapter 9	Resilience in youth after motor vehicle accidents *Mark S Barajas and Heath Schechinger*	177
Chapter 10	Post-Traumatic Stress Disorder and Motor Vehicle Crashes in Children and Adolescents: What Does the Future Hold? *Donald E Greydanus and Joav Merrick*	197

Section two: Acknowledgments		**205**
Chapter 11	About the editors	207
Chapter 12	About the Department of Pediatric and Adolescent Medicine, Western Michigan University Homer Stryker MD School of Medicine (WMED), Kalamazoo, Michigan, United States	211
Chapter 13	About the National Institute of Child Health and Human Development in Israel	215
Chapter 14	About the book series "Pediatrics, child and adolescent health"	219

Section three: Index	**223**
Index	225

DEDICATION

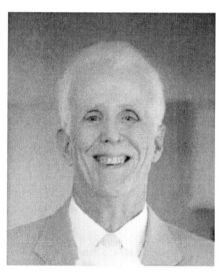

It is with great pleasure that this book is dedicated to Ross Gibson, MA in Counseling Psychology from Western Michigan University, as he has been a tremendous influence in my life professionally and personally. Ross gave me my first job as a psychologist shortly after graduating with my master's degree; taking a chance on someone with very little experience. During our work together Ross took me under his wing and exemplified professional and ethical behavior and was able to provide a strong foundation at the very beginning of my career; without such influence I would not be where I am today.

In addition to being a great mentor Ross is also a brilliant psychologist having trained under Aaron T Beck, MD (born 1921), professor emeritus at the Department of Psychiatry, University of Pennsylvania, in the use of cognitive behavioral therapy in New Hampshire in the 1980s. Ross also trained in dialectical behavioral therap, and has 40 years of experience in providing behavioral health services to children and adults in the community. For the last 15 years, he has provided treatment, with a focus on assaultive and sexual offenses, for adult male prisoners as a psychologist for the State of Michigan at the Charles Eger Reception and Guidance Center, where his current duties include suicide prevention screening upon admission to prison and making segregation rounds.

Ross has been a role model to countless trainees, employees, and friends at how to navigate the sometimes very complicated mental health work place all while maintaining personal dignity, respect for everyone and being able to continue to provide quality mental health services.

For those that know Ross, it goes without saying that he is a tireless advocate for equality for everyone. He is outspoken when it comes to fair and equal treatment for anyone who may have been discriminated against and never shies away from a controversial conversation if it is intended to help others. Such a quality is invaluable; particularly to a mental health professional.

Ross, it is my hope to carry on what you have taught me over the years with my trainees, employees, and all of the important people in my life. Thank you again for the example you have set.

Assistant professor Roger W Apple,
PhD, Pediatrics Psychology, Department of Pediatric and Adolescent
Medicine, Western Michigan University, Homer Stryker MD School of
Medicine, 1000 Oakland Drive, Kalamazoo, MI 49008-1284, United States.
Email: roger.apple@med.wmich.edu

PREFACE

First of all Donald E Greydanus dedicates this book to his grandchildren: Talus Everett, Gavriella Hazel Paige, John Elliot, Calvin Tibideau, Lucinda Joan Louise, Felix Mark, Graydon Samuel, Arje Donald, Emmett Christopher, Konrad Weston, and the unborn Californians. You have been and will be influenced by motor vehicles in the 21st century---now as passengers and pedestrians, but soon as drivers as well! Your Opa wishes you safety and joy in all these experiences! "ab imo pectore" (from the heart).

The first steam-powered vehicle is attributed to the Flemish Jesuit missionary Ferdinand Verbiest (1623-1688) in China and made in 1672 for the Chinese Emperor who was called the Kangxi Emperor (Enkh Amgalan Khaan (1654-1722)—the fourth emperor of the Qing dynasty) (1,2). A variety of engineers and others experimented with the concept of a vehicle propelled by steam in the 17th to 20th centuries and then electric automobiles and vehicles with internal combustion engines of the 20th and 21st centuries. Henry Ford (1863-1947) was the American industrialist who manufactured the famous Ford Model T (1908-1927) that was mass produced via the assembly line method that allowed middle class Americans to be able to buy their own automobiles (3).

The first recorded automobile death was Mary Ward in Ireland who was thrown from a steam-powered car and fell under its wheels in 1869. The first known automobile accident in a gasoline-powered vehicle in the United States was recorded in Ohio City, Ohio in 1891 with engineer James Lambert driving and hitting a tree root (4). History records the first person killed by an automobile accident in the United States as Henry Bliss (1830-1899) in New York City on September 13, 1899 (5). He was killed on a Wednesday and thus, this event did not contribute to triskaidekaphobia. A plaque was made and dedicated to Henry Bliss on September 13, 1999 in New York City:

> "Here at West 74th Street and Central Park West, Henry H. Bliss dismounted from a streetcar and was struck and knocked unconscious by an automobile on the evening of September 13, 1899. When Mr. Bliss, a New York real estate man, died the next morning from his injuries, he became the first recorded motor vehicle fatality in the Western Hemisphere. This sign was erected to remember Mr. Bliss on the centennial of his untimely death and to promote safety on our streets and highways" (6)

The number one cause of death for American youths is the motor vehicle crash (cars, motorcycles, all-terrain vehicles, others) (7,8). As the automobile became popular among humans, motor vehicle crashes became the major cause of death and disability among children and adolescents. Research initially focused on the physical trauma that motor crashes induced, but eventually the psychological toll of these crashes in the pediatric population became appreciated including the sequela of post-traumatic stress disorder (1).

This book "Children and youth: Post-traumatic stress disorder and motor vehicle crashes" explores various issues of this far-reaching problem in 21st century life. We look at a historical reflection from the 20th to the 21st century as society became more aware of post-traumatic stress disorder (PTSD) and vehicular crashes affecting the pediatric population, demographics including current as well as past national crash statistics, factors involved in dangerous driving, PTSD assessment concepts, PTSD differential diagnoses and comorbidities, psychological impact of PTSD, issues for teachers, PTSD and resilience, and management principles for PTSD. We conclude with potential concepts of future predictions, including the emerging role of artificial intelligence.

The editors thank the various experts in this manuscript for providing us with their invaluable time and expertise. The editors sincerely hope that the readers will benefit from the information presented in this publication and we thank the publisher, Nova Biomedical Science, for working with us to get this book out in print.

Founding Chair and Professor Donald E Greydanus,
MD, DrHC (Athens), Department of Pediatric and Adolescent Medicine, Western Michigan University, Homer Stryker MD School of Medicine, 1000

Oakland Drive, Kalamazoo, MI 49008-1284, United States. Email: Donald.greydanus@med.wmich.edu

Professor Joav Merrick, MD, MMedSci, DMSc, Medical Director, Health Services, Division for Intellectual and Developmental Disabilities, Ministry of Social Affairs and Social Services, POBox 1260, IL-91012 Jerusalem, Israel. Email: jmerrick@zahav.net.il

REFERENCES

[1] Greydanus DE, Merrick J. Post-traumatic stress disorder and motor vehicle accidents. J Pain Manage 2016; (1):3-7.
[2] Setright LJK. Drive on! A social history of the motor car. London: Granta Books, 2004.
[3] Ford H: My life and work: The autobiography of Henry Ford. New York: Barnes Noble, 1923.
[4] List of traffic collisions. URL: https://en.wikipedia.org/wiki/List_of_traffic_collisions.
[5] Bailey LS. 1881 Lambert: A new claim for America's first gasoline automobile. Antique Automobile 24.5. 1960:340-400.
[6] Henry H Bliss. URL: https://en.wikipedia.org/wiki/Henry_H._Bliss.
[7] Centers for Disease Control and Prevention. Youth Risk Behavior Surveillance, United States, 1997. MMWR 1998;47(SS-3):1-89.
[8] Rosen DS, Xiangdong M, Blum RW. Adolescent health: Current trends and critical issues. State Art Rev Adolesc Med 1990;1(1):15-31.

INTRODUCTION

In: Children and Youth
Editors: Donald E. Greydanus et al.
ISBN: 978-1-53611-102-6
© 2017 Nova Science Publishers, Inc.

Chapter 1

INTRODUCTION TO POST-TRAUMATIC STRESS DISORDER AND MOTOR VEHICLE CRASHES IN CHILDREN AND ADOLESCENTS: A HISTORICALLY DELAYED REALIZATION

Donald E Greydanus[1,*], *MD, DrHC(Athens)*
and Joav Merrick[2-6], *MD, MMedSci, DMSc*

[1]Department of Pediatric and Adolescent Medicine, Western Michigan University Homer Stryker MD School of Medicine, Kalamazoo, Michigan, United States, [2]National Institute of Child Health and Human Development, Jerusalem, Israel, [3]Health Services, Division for Intellectual and Developmental Disabilities, Ministry of Social Affairs and Social Services, Jerusalem, Israel, [4]Department of Pediatrics, Mt Scopus Campus, Hadassah Hebrew University Medical Center, Jerusalem, Israel, [5]Kentucky Children's Hospital, University of Kentucky, Lexington, Kentucky, United States and [6]Center for Healthy Development, School of Public Health, Georgia State University, Atlanta, US

The first steam-powered vehicle is attributed to Ferdinand Verbiest in China made in 1672 for the Kangxi Emperor. The first recorded automobile death was Mary Ward in Ireland who was thrown from a

---

[*] Correspondence: Donald E. Greydanus, MD, DrHC(Athens), Department of Pediatric and Adolescent Medicine, Western Michigan University Homer Stryker MD School of Medicine, Kalamazoo, MI 49008-1284, United States. E-mail: Donald.greydanus@med.wmich.edu.

steam-powered car and fell under its wheels in 1869. The first person killed in the United States is recorded as Henry Bliss in New York City on Wednesday, September 13, 1899. As the automobile became popular among all groups of humans, motor vehicle crashes became the major cause of death and disability among children and adolescents. Research initially focused on the physical trauma that motor vehicle accidents or crashes induced, but eventually the psychological toll of motor vehicle crashes (MVCs) in the pediatric population became appreciated. This discussion reflects on how this occurred taking the entire 20th century to be acknowledged by researchers, clinicians, parents, and the general society.

"The modern motor vehicles are safer and more reliable than they have ever been – yet more than 1 million people are killed in accidents around the world each year and more than 50 million are injured. Why? Largely because of a perilous element in the mechanics of driving remains unperfected by progress: the human being."

Tom Chatfield (British author, born in 1980)

INTRODUCTION

The first steam-powered vehicle is attributed to Ferdinand Verbiest in China made in 1672 for the Chinese Emperor who was called the Kangxi Emperor (Enkh Amgalan Khaan—the fourth emperor of the Qing dynasty (1, 2). A variety of engineers and others experimented with the concept of a vehicle propelled by steam in the 17th to 20th centuries and then electric automobiles and vehicles with internal combustion engines of the 20th and 21st centuries. Henry Ford (1863-1947) was the American industrialist who manufactured the famous Ford Model T (1908-1927) that was mass produced via the assembly line method that allowed middle class Americans to be able to buy their own automobiles (3).

The first recorded automobile death was Mary Ward in Ireland who was in an automobile accident in a gasoline-powered vehicle in 1869 (4). The first recorded motor vehicle accident in the United States was in Ohio City, Ohio in 1891; engineer James Lambert was driving and he hit a tree root (5). History records the first person killed by an automobile accident in the United States was Henry Bliss (1830-1899) in New York City on September 13, 1899 (6). He was killed on a Wednesday and thus, this event did not contribute to triskaidekaphobia. A plaque was made and dedicated to Henry Bliss on September 13, 1999 in New York City:

> "Here at West 74th Street and Central Park West, Henry H. Bliss dismounted from a streetcar and was struck and knocked unconscious by an automobile on the evening of September 13, 1899. When Mr. Bliss, a New York real estate man, died the next morning from his injuries, he became the first recorded motor vehicle fatality in the Western Hemisphere. This sign was erected to remember Mr. Bliss on the centennial of his untimely death and to promote safety on our streets and highways" (6)

COMPLEXITIES OF MOTOR VEHICLE CRASHES (MVCS)

Perhaps billions of persons have driven motor vehicles over the past century and this has resulted in countless traffic accidents, injuries, and deaths since the days of Mary Ward in Ireland, James Lambert in Ohio, and Henry Bliss of New York City. Children and adolescents are involved in these deaths and injuries in various ways both as pedestrians and passengers, while adolescents may also be part of this risk scenario as drivers of motor vehicles. For example, in the 21st century there are approximately 900 pedestrians killed by MVCs who are under age 19 years along with 51,000 who are injured; approximately 5,300 of these pediatric persons are hospitalized each year because of MVCs in the United States (7).

Motor vehicle crashes are the number one cause of death for children ages 4 years and older (8). The US Fatality Analysis Reporting System is a registry of motor vehicles deaths across the United States and a review of its 1991 to 1996 data reveals that 16,676 children under 16 years of age were killed as passengers, pedestrians, or bicyclists because of a motor vehicle crash; nearly 20% of these deaths involved crashes in which alcohol was involved (9). A review of the United States 2001-2010 Fatality Analysis Reporting System (FARS) data notes that 2,344 children under age 15 years of age were killed in motor vehicle crashes that involved at least one driver who was alcohol-impaired; 65% were in the car of an alcohol-impaired driver (i.e., blood alcohol concentration of =0.08 g/dL (10).

Approximately 75% of deaths in in American youth (ages 14 to 24 years of age) resulted from four causes: motor vehicle accidents, other unintentional injuries, homicide, and suicide (11). Motor vehicle accidents account for 30%

of these deaths and are the number one cause of death in this age group (11). An important cause of these deaths is the inexperience with driving skills that youth often possess along with increased risk taking behavior, dangerous driving patterns (such as excessive speed), and drug-impaired driving (i.e., alcohol, cannabis, others) (11-14).

All-terrain vehicles (ATV) deaths occur as well as noted by a study from 2007 to 2011 of the Fatality Analysis Reporting System that revealed 1,701 ATV fatalities (15). The high death rate of crashes involving adolescent and young adult driving motorcycles remains of concern as well because of reckless driving behavior, lack of helmets, use of drugs, and other factors (16). In 2010 there were 3,951 reported deaths from motorcycle accidents in the United States in which 77% died at the accident scene, 10% died in the emergency department, and 13% died in the hospital; 69% of the deaths involved persons not wearing a helmet (17). Modern means of transportation means that a number of vehicle accidents can occur, such as a bus-train collision that can result in severe psychiatric consequences to the survivors who can be children (18).

The price families and society pay for each of these deaths is beyond comprehension. Also troubling is that for every death in these tragic accidents, there are many more who are injured and face a potential lifetime of disability. Motor vehicle crashes remain a leading cause of not only death, but also disability in children and youth in the United States (19). Historically, recognition of potential psychological problems after car crashes emerged very slowly in the 20th century Western medicine (20-22). MVC-related personal injury litigation is a complex phenomenon, called by some experts as a "forensic minefield" that has crossed from the 20th to the 21st century (23).

MVA-RELATED PTSD IN CHILDREN AND YOUTH

There was some early recognition in England regarding potential psychological problems related to being involved in motor vehicle crashes. Miller commented on what was called "accident neurosis" in 1961 and a 1985 study by Tarsh and Royston provided a study looking at this condition (24-26).

In 1992 HL Freeman, editor of the British Journal of Psychiatry, sent a letter to the Journal of the Royal Society of Medicine (London, England) commenting on a paper published in this journal dealing with the high cost of traffic accidents that society must face; in his letter, HL Freeman pointed out that the article did not mention "the psychiatric consequences of RTAs" (road traffic accidents) and that "there is a scarcity of reliable data on these sequelae (27)." He also noted that the psychological effects of these accidents were consistent with post-traumatic stress disorder. He noted that there was limited data except for the study by Tarsh and Royston and did not agree with the "accident neurosis" term (27). In 1993 Thompson and associates sent a letter to the British Medical Journal commenting on an article dealing with psychiatric morbidity in adults injuries in MVAs and astutely pointing out that "….morbidity is also important in children (28)."

EARLY COMMENTS FROM NORTH AMERICA

Research on MVAs in the United States began to be published in the middle of the 20th century focusing on orthopedic injuries in adults and some recognition of these injuries in children began to appear in the 1970s in North America (29-32). However, it was not until the penultimate decade of the 20th century that astute appreciation arose for the psychological nature of injuries that were an important part of the sequelae of MVAs in children and adults.

PTSD AND MVAS: RESEARCH FINALLY OCCURS IN CHILDREN IN THE 20TH CENTURY

It was in 1980 that the American Psychiatric Association added the term, posttraumatic stress disorder, to its lexicon of mental disorders---the DSM III or Diagnostic and Statistical Manual of Mental Disorders (33, 34). The basis of posttraumatic stress disorder (PTSD) was that trauma can lead to repeated experience of the traumatic event with symptoms of augmented arousal and attempts to avoid these unpleasant symptoms (34). The link of PTSD and car accidents was seen with the 1981 publication of Walker who also discussed methods of treatment (22). As the last decade of the 20th century marched on, researchers and clinicians came to the gradual realization that the nature of trauma experienced in motor vehicle accidents (MVA) can lead to posttraumatic stress disorder (PTSD) as well as other psychiatric consequences (i.e., anxiety, depression) in some of those that are involved (34-39).

Stimulated by the comments of British scholars in the early 1990s (27, 28), researchers began to unravel connections between MVC and PTSD in children and adolescents. One group looked at 25 adolescents involved in a school-related MVA in the Austrian Alps and in 1996, concluded that psychological outcomes were worse for the girls versus the boys and for those who were hospitalized as a result of their injuries (40). This raised the issue of seeking any correlation between the severity of the physical injury and the severity of the psychological sequelae—a topic researched later in the 21st century. This report also noted that psychological problems can continue long after the accident and after fractures have healed.

In a 1997 study Di Gallo et al. interviewed 57 young victims of car accidents aged 5 to 18 years of age and their parents; these interviews occurred at 2-16 days and 12-15 weeks after the accident (41). Symptoms of stress were seen at both interviews but less at the second one; at the end 14% of the young victims had moderate or severe PTSD while 17% had serious traffic-related fear and parents also noted post-accident mood disturbances (41).

Another group published a 12 month prospective study in 1998 that studied 119 children (ages 5-18 years) and compared them to 66 children who had sports injuries (42). They found PTSD in 34.5% of the children involved in MVCs versus 3% in those with sports injuries. They noted that PTSD was identified in one-third of the MVC victims six weeks after their trauma and that the psychological needs of these children remained "largely unrecognized." This set the stage for more research into the 21st century.

Another British study reported on a consecutive sample of 8 to 16 year olds involved in a motor vehicle accident who were interviewed 6 weeks and 6 months after their accidents (43). Criteria for PTSD (DSM-IV, 1994) were seen in 75% and symptoms found included major depressive disorder and anxiety disorders. Six months after their MVC, 17% continued with PTSD symptoms (43). Factors that seemed to increase chances for the development of PTSD were noted as being female, MVC involvement, and pre-existing mental illness (i.e, anxiety, depression) (43).

Another European study published in 1998 looked at 45 school age children who had been involved in road traffic accidents and who did not have specific head trauma (44). Questionnaire-derived data noted that short-term psychological sequelae were common, one-third had moderately severe problems 4-7 months post-accident, and 11% were severely affected. Parents noted travel anxiety, depression, generalized anxiety, sleep problems, irritability, and anger. Those most at risk for psychological sequelae were young children, children who had not recovered from their physical injuries, and those whose parent(s) were also injured (44).

A prospective cohort study of children ages 3 to 18 years of age was published in the American literature in 1999 (45). These victims (children and parents) of MVCs were given a validated questionnaire at 7 to 12 months post-injury. Diagnostic PTSD was noted in 25% of the children and 15% of the parents; only 46% of the parents sought professional help for their children and only 20% of the affected parents sought such help (45). Precipitating factors for the child having PTSD was being an older child and having a parent with PTSD; an important factor for parent PTDS was having witnessed the accident of their child.

As the 20th century drew to a close, acknowledgment of the existence of MVC-related PTSD in children and adolescents had grown setting the stage for further research in the 21st century. It took over 130 years from the first known death in Ireland from a MVC for the realization to occur that our romance with the motorized vehicle has cost society dearly in terms of not only physical trauma, but psychological trauma to millions of our children and youth. This should cause some further pedagogical reflections of effects of the motorized vehicles on our beloved children as well as ways to prevent these accidents and their negative effects. History teaches us to use its lessons to focus on improving safety for our children and society, though risks will always be present (46). However, implementation of these lessons can be difficult and complex. Murphy, for example, noted in 1998 that potentially protective car seats can be used incorrectly and air bags may result in the death of children (47). Perhaps more protective lessons can be learned in the 21st century to protect children, adolescents, and adults from the potential devastation of motor vehicle crashes (MVCs)

LESSONS FROM THE 21ST CENTURY SO FAR

The 20th century finally introduced the potential link between MVCs and the anxiety syndrome called PTSD in children and adolescents. Such work stimulated continued research into the complex relationships and underpinnings between MVCs and PTSD. For example, research early in this decade on 43 children and their parents 6 weeks after a traffic accident noted that PTSD can occur in those with and without mild traumatic brain injury (TBI) and mild TBI did not influence the risk for PTSD in this population (48). However, later research reported findings of more white matter abnormalities in persons who survived PTSD and developed PTSD versus MVC persons who did not develop PTSD (49).

Research notes that head trauma with loss of consciousness in MVCs increases the risks for developing PTSD (50). Current studies also suggest that brain-derived neurotrophic factor (protein that is found in the neurotrophic group of growth factors) may be protective for PTSD if found in sufficiently high levels (51). Also of interest is the findings of neural changes in the anterior cingulate cortex (ACC) of those with PTSD; the ACC is a cerebral structure involved in mechanisms of fear-conditioning (52).

Studies in this decade noted that any child involved in MVCs can develop PTDS and an important key in this development is the presence of peri-traumatic distress (53, 54). Some persons appear to be more susceptible to PTSD than others based on genetic predisposition, the nature of the trauma event, and other factors (55). In these persons a variety of posttraumatic psychological sequelae may arise that include PTSD, depression, anxiety, others (56). In adults with post-MVA PTSD, this psychological disorder is worse in drivers who feel the accident was their fault and/or who sustained serious injury (57).

Studies are looking at the posttraumatic nightmares of children with PTSD and their relationship to psychopathology (58). Studies note that factors which may involve the child in chronic PTSD after injury include psychological problems prior to the trauma, perceived threat to one's life, parental PTSD, and other factors (59). The study of the peri-trauma period is occurring which improves knowledge of the impact of trauma on the child based on improved knowledge of peri-traumatic distress that includes potential peri-traumatic guilt (60-62). Cost of caring for patients with PTSD is high, even higher than that seen with controls having major depressive disorder (MDD) (63).

PTSD EVALUATION

Tools for assessment of PTSD continue to be developed such as seen with the Clinician Administered Post-traumatic Scale for Children (CAPS-C) that has been used in England to identify post-traumatic depression (Birleson Depression Inventory), anxiety (Revised Manifest Anxiety Scale), and coping style (Kidcope) (64). Another scale that has been developed is the 36-item observer-report instrument called the Child Stress Disorders Checklist used in various settings to identify acute stress disorder (ASD) and PTSD in children (65).

Others include the Child Behavior Checklist (CBCL), the Screening Tool for Early Predictors of PTSD (STEPP), the Pediatric Emotional Distress Scale (PEDS), the Pediatric Emotional Distress Scale Early Screener (PEDS-ES), and the Children's Revised Impact of Event Scale (CRIES) with two versions

(CRIES-8, CRIES-13) (66-69). Research during this decade also concluded that modification of screening tools for PTSD must occur when evaluating young children involved in motor vehicle crashes (70). Surveys or scales may also be useful in assessing aspects of treatment in PTSD such as the use of the Driving Behavior Survey (DBS) to assess the effect of treatment in anxious driving behavior in those with PTSD who are old enough to drive (71).

DSM-5 AND PTSD

The American Psychiatric Association's DSM-III was published in 1980, the DSM-III-IV in 1987, and DSM-IV in 1994, the DSM-IV-TR in 2000, and the latest DSM—DSM-5--in May of 2013 (72). Changes to PTSD were made in the 2013 version including reclassifying this condition from an anxiety disorder to a new chapter: Trauma and Stressor-Related disorders. Controversy exists with these changes and thus, when reviewing research on PTSD, one needs to know what definitions the authors are using (73, 74).

ASD AND PTSD LINKS

Studies in this decade also looked at links between acute stress disorder (ASD) and PTSD after MVCs (75). The development of post-trauma ASD is not always a good or optimal predictor of the development of PTSD (75, 76). Dissociation appears to be more important in ASD than in PTSD (77, 78). Though clinicians who treat children typically underestimate PTSD in children, it is important for all clinicians to understand that even young children can develop PTSD as well as ASD, that they may continue to worry about future harm after their accident, and that direct interviews are needed in children exposed to MVCs (79-81). ASD and PTSD are complex issues requiring further study in children and adolescents exposed to MVCs.

NEUROENDOCRINE LINKS WITH PTSD

Studies in this decade provided further evidence for neuroendocrine underpinnings in PTSD noting that PTSD symptoms can be due to trauma-induced changes in the hypothalamic-pituitary-adrenal (HPA) axis and the noradrenergic system (82, 83). A number of brain components are involved in this process including the hippocampus (subcortical), amygdala (located within the temporal lobes), and locus coeruleus (locus coeruleus-noradrenergic system). The locus coeruleus is a nucleus in the brainstem structure called the pons and is associated with human responses to panic and stress (82).

Trauma leads to alterations in these structures, systems and HPA axis that induces lower cortical levels, heightened glucocorticoid receptors' reactions, and alterations in the HPA negative feedback inhibition (82). Plasma noradrenaline levels can in increased as well as heart rates in those with posttraumatic stress syndrome (84, 85). Greek researchers have documented a progressive divergence of noradrenaline and cortisol levels seen in children after MVCs (84). Also, research suggests that these trauma-induced changes in neuroendocrine function at critical times in the brain development may have permanent effects on behavioral maturation (86, 87).

Perhaps teaching clinicians the neuroendocrine abnormalities that induce PTSD may encourage more early recognition of this condition that can arise after MVCs in 25% to 33% of children and adolescents (58). This is especially important in view of research that notes PTSD can be delayed in children prompting a recommendation to monitor these young patients for weeks after an MVC for the potential development of PTSD (88).

PTSD MANAGEMENT

Research concludes that treatment of PTSD should begin early and be comprehensive to help the pediatric patient and the family. A team approach may be useful utilizing various clinicians experienced in both the physiologic and psychological impact of trauma. Clinicians should take a proactive stance and contact the family 7 to 14 days after the motor vehicle crash (MVC) to ask about potential psychological features in the injured child or adolescent (89). Experts conclude that the more support given to these persons the better their outcomes will be (90). A visit to the office may be useful to elicit more data including potential negative effects on the family. Such a step is also important for children who have been hit by a motor vehicle as they are at risk for PTSD and their parents may be at more risk for these symptoms than parents whose child was in a motor vehicle accident per se (89). Even with so-called "mild" physical injury, those with PTSD have reduced quality of life (QOL) (91-95).

Anticipatory guidance is important for families involved in MVCs though the precise benefits of therapy is not clear at this time (96-98). A variety of therapies are utilized for these patients and their families with the best results seen with cognitive-behavioral therapy (99). Parents with psychopathology (i.e., trait anxiety) increase the risk for their post-MVC child to develop PTSD and thus, treatment of the parent may help with issues of PTSD in the child (100). The development of trait anxiety in the post-MVC person suggests the development of a more severe PTSD (101).

The use of psychopharmacology has not produced clearly beneficial results and more research is need in this area as well as in the overall benefit of psychological therapies especially with the lack of research demonstrating long-term benefit with chronic PTSD (59, 102, 103). Though the use of hydrocortisone may have some benefit in adults for prevention of PTSD, those receiving benzodiazepines tended to have higher prevalence of PTSD (104, 105). Use of thought control strategies for dealing with intrusive PTSD symptoms has not been shown to be effective in youth (106).

PTSD OUTCOMES

Children and adolescents who develop PTSD after a MVC demonstrate repeated encounters with feelings from the traumatic events with autonomic hyperarousal and seek to avoid factors that stimulate these feelings (82). Studies suggest that chronic PTSD may develop despite attempts with cognitive-behavioral therapy to alleviate the impact of this condition even in young children (107,108). These individuals can develop anger, depression, alienation from other persons, effects on philosophy of life, and various comorbid conditions (i.e., anxiety, sleep dysfunction, attention dysfunction, conduct behavior, and learning difficulties) (109-114). Travel anxiety is common for these children and adolescents (115). MVCs in the 21st century contributes to depression, alcohol abuse, increased medication (for example, analgesics), and interpersonal violence in youth who have been involved in MVCs (116, 117). The potential for chronicity in negative psychological reactions including disruption in quality of life from MVCs necessitates the need for on-going therapy for these victims that includes cognitive-behavioral therapy and trauma-focused interventions (107, 108, 118).

CONCLUSION

Though death from a motor vehicle was recorded as early as 1869 in Ireland and 1899 in the United States, it took many decades for researchers, clinicians, and society to appreciate the dangers of driving a motor vehicle. The general public has had a great romance with the automobile since Henry Ford presented his famous Ford Model T (1908-1927) that eventually introduced the thrill of expanded transportation for billions of persons—whether one was wealthy or was the common person.

The impact of posttraumatic stress disorder occurring after MVCs was studied in the 20th century and was part of this century's study of the effects of trauma in general on human beings stimulated by the tragic effects of World War II in the Netherlands and other countries in the 21st century (119-122). Research on post-MVC PTSD has taught us that this disorder can arise from a variety of traumas including assault (or threat of violence), being in an intensive care unit for illness or injury, near drowning, humiliation by others, attempted suicide, and others (123).

In this discussion some of the complex data on these accidents have been reviewed for drivers, passengers, and pedestrians. Initially only the physical (ie, orthopedic) aftermath of motor vehicle crashes were studied and appreciated by the middle of the 20th century. The introduction of the term posttraumatic stress disorder in 1980 allowed British scholars to alert others to a potential link between MVCs and PTSD in the 1990s. This set the stage for more formal research on adults and then on children as well as adolescents. Some of this late 20th century and early 21st century research is reviewed as it pertains to the pediatric population. The data being accumulated should allow society to pause and carefully consider how we can protect our children of the 21st century from the potential dangers of motor vehicle accidents (124). Various concepts of motor vehicle crashes (often called motor vehicle accidents in earlier literature) and PTSD are also considered in other parts of this publication. The motor vehicle crash can be considered part of the overall phenomenon of childhood violence that cries out for a change in social norms to avoid being accepted as simply inevitable normal death in our children (125).

"To be ignorant of what occurred before you were born is to remain always a child. For what is the worth of human life, unless it is woven into the life of our ancestors by the records of history."

Marcus Tullius Cicero (106 BC to 43 BC)

REFERENCES

[1] Greydanus DE, Merrick J. Post-traumatic stress disorder and motor vehicle accidents. J Pain Manage 2016;9(1):3-7.
[2] Setright LJK. Drive on! A social history of the motor car. London: Granta Books, 2004.
[3] Ford H: My life and work: The autobiography of Henry Ford. New York: Barnes Noble, 1923.
[4] List of traffic collisions. URL: https://en.wikipedia.org/wiki/List_of_traffic_collisions.
[5] Bailey LS. 1881 Lambert: A new claim for America's first gasoline automobile. Antique Automobile 1960;24(5):340-400.
[6] Henry H Bliss. URL: https://en.wikipedia.org/wiki/Henry_H._Bliss.
[7] Committee on Injury, Violence, and Poison Prevention. American Academy of Pediatrics Policy statement: Pdestrian safety. Pediatrics 2009;124(2):802-12.
[8] Durbin DR. Committee on Injury, Violence, and Poison Prevention. Pediatrics 2011;127(4):e1050-66.
[9] Margolis LH, Foss FD, Tolbert WG. Alcohol and motor vehicle-related deaths of children as passengers, pedestrians, and bicyclists. JAMA 2000;283(17):2245-8.
[10] Quinlan K, Shults RA, Rudd RA. Child passenger deaths involving alcohol-impaired drivers. Pediatrics 2014;133(6):966-72.
[11] Patel DR. Greydanus DE, Rowlett JD. Romance with the automobile in the 20th century: implications for adolescents in a new millennium. Adolesc Med 2000;11(1):127-39.
[12] Greydanus DE, Kaplan G, Baxter LE Sr., Patel DR, Feucht CL. Cannabis: The never-ending, nefarious nepenthe of the 21st century: what should the clinician know? Dis Mon 2015;61(4):118-75.
[13] Gonzales MM, Dickinson LM, DiGuiseppi C, Lowenstein SR. Student drivers: a study of fatal motor vehicle crashes involving 16-year-old drivers. Ann Emerg Med 2005;45(2):140-6.
[14] Shope JT, Bingham CR. Teen driving: motor-vehicle crashes and factors that contribute. Am J Prev Med 2008;35(3 Suppl):S261-71.
[15] Williams AF, Oesch SL, McCartt AT, Teoh ER, Sims LB. On-road-all-terrain vehicle (ATV) fatalities in the United States. J Safety Res 2014;50:117-23.
[16] Jung S, Xiao Q, Yoon Y. Evaluation of motorcycle safety strategies using the severity of injuries. Accid Anal Prev 2013;59:357-64.
[17] Dua A, Wei S, Safarik J, Furlough C, Desai SS. National mandatory motorcycle helmet laws may save $2.2 billion annually: an inpatient and value of statistical life analysis. J Trauma Acute Care Surg 2015;78(6):1182-6.
[18] Tyano S, Iancu I, Solomon Z, Sever J, Goldstein I, Touviana Y, et al. Seven-year follow-up of child survivors of a bus-train collision. J Am Acad Child Adolesc Psychiatry 1996;35(3):365-73.
[19] Murphy JM. Child passenger safety. J Pediatr Health Care 1998;12(3):130-8.
[20] Wilson WP, Hohman LB, Workman SN. Psychiatric sequelae of automobile accidents. NC Med J 1965;26(10):453-7.

[21] Culpan R, Taylor C. Psychiatric disorders following road traffic and industrial injuries. Aust NZ J Psychiatry 1973;7(1):32.
[22] Walker JI. Posttraumatic stress disorder after a car accident. Postgrad Med 1981;69(2):82,84,86.
[23] Sparr LF, Boehnlein JK. Posttraumatic stress disorder in tort actions: forensic minefield. Bull Am Acad Psychiatry Law 1990;18(3):283-302.
[24] Miller H. Accident neurosis Part 1 & 2. BMJ 1961;1:919-25;992.
[25] Tarsh MJE, Royston C. A follow-up of accident neurosis. Br J Psychiatry 1985;146:18-25.
[26] Freeman HL. The cost of traffic casualties to the community. (Letter). J R Soc Med 1992;85(2):121-2.
[27] Thompson A, McArdle P. Dunne F. Psychiatric consequences of road traffic accidents. Children may also be seriously affected. (Letter). BMJ 1993;307(6914):1282-3.
[28] Robertson RC. The automobile accident victim and skeletal injuries. Bull Am Coll Surg 1955;40(6):516-9.
[29] Anderson MX. Injuries caused by motor vehicles; a statistical analysis. Calif Med 1957;86(2):115-8.
[30] Reed MH. Pelvic fractures in children. J Can Assoc Radiol 1976;27(4):255-61.
[31] Cumming DC, Wren FD. Fetal skull fracture from an apparently trivial motor vehicle accident. Am J Obstet Gynecol 1978;132(3):342-3.
[32] American Psychiatric Association. Diagnostic and statistical manual of mental disorders, 3rd Edition (DSM III). Washington, DC: APA, 1980.
[33] Van der Kolk B. Posttraumatic stress disorder and the nature of trauma. Dialogues Clin Neurosci 2000;2(1):7-22.
[34] Blanchard EB, Hickling EJ, Barton KA, Taylor AE, Loos WR, Jones-Alexander J. One-year prospective follow-up of motor vehicle accident victims. Behav Res Ther 1996;34(10):775-86.
[35] Fearnley D. Psychological consequences of road accidents in children and adolescents. Br J Psychiatry 1997;171:393.
[36] Mayou R, Bryant B, Duthie R. Psychiatric consequences of road traffic accidents. BMJ 1993;307(6905):647-51.
[37] Mayou R, Tyndel S, Bryant B. Long-term outcome of motor vehicle accident injury. Psychosom Med 1997;59(6):578-84.
[38] Tonkin R. One adolescent's injury—a continuing saga. Inj Prev 1999;5(2):88-9.
[39] Curle CE, Williams C. Post-traumatic stress reactions in children: gender differences in the incidence of trauma reactions at two years and examination of factors influencing adjustment. Br J Clin Psychol 1996;35(Pt 2):297-309.
[40] Stallard P, Velleman R, Baldwin S. Prospective study of post-traumatic stress disorder in children involved in road traffic accidents. BMJ 1998;317(7173):1619-23.
[41] Di Gallo A, Barton J, Parry-Jones WL. Road traffic accidents: early psychological consequences in children and adolescents. Br J Psychiatry 1997;170(4):358-362.
[42] Mirza KA, Bhadrinath BR, Goodyer IM, Gilmour C. Post-traumatic stress disorder in children and adolescents following road traffic accidents. Br J Psychiatry 1998;172:443-7.

[43] Ellis A, Stores G, Mayou R. Psychological consequences of road traffic accidents in children. Eur Child Adolesc Psychiatry 1998;7(2):61-8.
[44] De Vries AP, Kassam-Adams N, Cnaan A, Sherman-Slate E, Gallagher PR, Winston FK. Looking beyond the physical injury; Post-traumatic stress disorder in children and parents after pediatric traffic injury. Pediatrics 1999;104(6):1293-9.
[45] Weatherwax M, Coddington J, Ahmed A, Richards EA. Child passenger safety policy and guidelines: Why change is imperative. J Pediatr Heatlh Care 2015 oct 27. pii: S0891-5245(15)00305-3.
[46] Diels C, Bos JE. Self-driving carsickness. Appl Ergon 2016;53(Pt B):374-382.
[47] Murphy JM, Child passenger safety. J Pediatr Health Care 1998;12(3):130-8.
[48] Mather FJ, Tate RL, Hannan TJ. Post-traumatic stress disorder in children following road traffic accidents: a comparison of those with and without mild traumatic brain injury. Brain Inj 2003;17(12):1077-87.
[49] Hu H, Zhou Y, Wang Q, Su S, Qiu Y, Ge J, et al. Association of abnormal white matter integrity in the acute phase of motor vehicle accidents with post-traumatic stress disorder. J Affect Disord 2016;190:714-22.
[50] Roitman P, Gilad M, Ankri YL, Shalev AY. Head injury and loss of consciousness raise the likelihood of developing and maintaining PTSD symptoms. J Trauma Stress 2013;26(6):727-34.
[51] Su S, Xiao Z, Lin Z, Qui Y, Jin Y, Wang Z. Plasma-brain derived neurotrophic factor levels in patients suffering from post-traumatic stress disorder. Psychiatr Res 2015;229(1-2):365-9.
[52] Boccia M, Piccardi L, Cordellieri P, Guariglia C, Giannini AM. EMDR therapy after motor vehicle accidents: meta-analystic evidence for specific treatment. Front Hum Neurosci 2015 Apr 21. doi: 10.3389/fnhum.2015.00213
[53] Olofsson E, Bunketorp O, Andersson AL. Children and adolescents injured in traffic-associated psychological consequences: a literature review. Acta Paediatr 2009;98(1):17-22.
[54] Bui E, Brunet A, Allenou C, Camassel C, Raynaud JP, Claudet I, et al. Peritraumatic reactions and posttraumatic stress symptoms in school-aged children victims of road traffic accidents. Gen Hosp Psychiatry 2010; 32(3): 330-3.
[55] Auxéméy Y. Posttraumatic stress disorder (PTSD) as a consequence of the interaction between an individual genetic susceptibility, a traumatogenic event and a social context. Encephale 2012;38(5):373-80. [French]
[56] Tierens M, Bal S, Crombez G, Van de Vorde P, Rosseel Y, Antrop I et al. The traumatic impact of motor vehicle accidents in high school students. J Pediatr Psychol 2012;37(1):1-10.
[57] Nickerson A, Aderka IM, Bryant RA, Hofmann SG. The role of attribution of trauma responsibility in posttraumatic stress disorder following motor vehicle accidents. Depress Anxiety 2013;30(5):483-8.
[58] Wittman L, Zehnder D, Schredl M, Jenni OG, Landolt MA. Posttraumatic nightmares and psychopathology in children after road traffic accidents. J Trauma Stress 2010;23(2):232-9.

[59] Kassam-Adams N, Marsac ML, Hildenbrand A, Winston FK. Postraumatic stress following pediatric injury: update on diagnosis, risk factors, and intervention. JAMA Pediatr 2013;167(12):1158-65.
[60] Marsac ML, Kassam-Adams N, Delahanty DL, Widaman KF, Barakat LP. Posttraumatic stress following acute medical trauma in children: a proposed model of bio-psycho-social processes during the peri-trauma period. Clin Child Fam Psychol Rev 2014;17(4):399-411.
[61] Lewis GC, Platts-Mills TF, Liberzon I, Bair E, Swor R, Peak D, et al. Incidence and predictors of acute psychological distress and dissociation after motor vehicle collision: a cross-sectional study. J Trauma Dissociation 2014;15(5):527-47.
[62] Haag AC, Zehnder D, Landolt MA. Guilt is associated with acute stress symptoms in children after road traffic accidents. Eur J Psychotraumatol 2015;6:29074. doi: 10.3402/ejpt.v6.29074.
[63] Ivanova JI, Birnbaum HG, Chen L, Duhig AM, Dayoub EJ, Kantor ES, et al. Cost of post-traumatic stress disorder vs major depressive disorder among patients covered by Medicaid or private insurance. Am J Manag Cost 2011;17(8):e314-23.
[64] Stallard P, Velleman R, Langsford J, Baldwin S. Coping and psychological distress in children involved in road traffic accidents. Br J Clin Psychol 2001;40(Pt 2):197-208.
[65] Saxe G, Chawla N, Stoddard F, Kassam-Adams N, Courtney D, Cunningham K, Lopez C et al. Child stress disorders checklist: a measure of ASD and PTDS in children. J Am Acad Child Adolesc Psychiatr 2003;42(8):972-8.
[66] Winston FK, Kassam-Adams N, Garcia-España F, Ittenback R, Cnaan A. Screening for risk of persistent posttraumatic stress in injured children and their parents. JAMA 2003;290(3):643-9.
[67] Kramer DN, Herti MB, Landolt MA. Evaluation of an early risk screener for PTSD in preschool children after accidental injury. Pediatrics 2013;132(4):e945-51.
[68] Dow BL, Kenardy JA, Le Brocque RM, Long DA. The utility of the Children's Revised Impact of Event Scale in screening for concurrent PTSD following admission to intensive care. J Trauma Stress 2012;25(5):602-5.
[69] van Meijel EP, Gigengack MR, Verlinden E, Opmeer BC, Heil HA, Goslings JC. et al. Predicting posttraumatic stress disorder in children and parents following accidental child injury: evaluation of the Screening Tool for Early Predictors of Posttraumatic Stress Disorder (STEPP). BMC Psychiatry 2015;15:113. doi: 10.1186/s12888-015-0492-z.
[70] Meiser-Stedman R, Smith P, Glucksman E, Yule W, Dalgieish T. The posttraumatic stress disorder diagnosis in preschool- and elementary school-age children exposed to motor vehicle accidents. Am J Psychiatry 2008;165(10):1326-37.
[71] Baker AS, Litwack SD, Clapp JD, Beck G, Sloan DM. The driving behavior survey as a measure of behavioral stress responses to MVA-related PTSD. Behav Ther 2014;45(3):444-53.
[72] American Psychiatric Association. Diagnostic and statistical manual of mental disorders, fifth edition. Arlington, VA: American Psychiatric Association, 2013.
[73] Shorter E. The history of nosology and the rise of the Diagnostic and Statistical Manual of Mental Disorders. Dialogues Clin Neurosci 2015;17(1):59-67.

[74] Stevens A, Fabra M. Forensic assessment of DSM-5 posttraumatic stress disorder: a commentary on the transition from DSM-IV-TR. Versicherungsmedizin 2013;65(4):191-6. [German]
[75] Kassam-Adams N, Winston FK. Predicting child PTSD: the relationship between acute stress disorder and PTSD in children. J Am Acad Child Adolesc Psychiatry 2004;43(4):403-11.
[76] Meisser-Stedman R, Yule W, Smith P, Glucksman E, Dalgleish T. Acute stress disorder and posttraumatic stress disorder in children and adolescents involved in assaults or motor vehicle accidents. Am J Psychiatry 2005;162(7):1381-3.
[77] Meisser-Stedman R, Dalgleish T, Smith P, Yule W, Glucksman E. Diagnostic, demographic, memory, quality, and cognitive variables associated with acute stress disorder in children and adolescents. J Abnorm Psychol 2007;116(1):65-79.
[78] Dalgleish T, Meisser-Stedman R, Kassam-Adams N, Ehlers A, Winston FK, Smith P et al. Predictive validity of acute stress disorder in children and adolescents. Br J Psychiatry 2008;192(5):392-3.
[79] Ziegler MF, Greenwald MH, De Guzman MA, Simon HK. Posttraumatic stress responses in children: awareness and practice among a sample of pediatric emergency care providers. Pediatrics 2005;115(5):1261-7.
[80] Meisser-Stedman R, Smith P, Glucksman E, Yule W, Dalgleish T. Parent and child agreement for acute stress disorder, post-traumatic stress disorder and other psychopathology in a prospective study of children and adolescents exposed to single-event trauma. J Abnorm Child Psychol 2007;35(2):191-201.
[81] Bryant RA, Salmon K, Sinclair E, Davidson P. A prospective study of appraisals in childhood posttraumatic stress disorder. Behav Res Ther 2007;45(10):2502-7.
[82] Birmes P, Escande M, Gourdy P, Schmitt L. Biological factors of post-traumatic stress: neuroendocrine aspects. Encephale 2000;26(6):55-61. [French]
[83] Langeland W, Olff M. Psychobiology of posttraumatic stress disorder in pediatric injury patients: a review of the literature. Neurosci Biobehav Rev 2008;32(1):161-74.
[84] Pervanidou P, Kolaitis G, Charitaki S, Lazaropoulou C, Papassotiriou I, Hindmarsh P, et al. The natural history of neuroendocrine changes in pediatric posttraumatic stress disorder (PTSD) after motor vehicle accidents: progressive divergence of noradrenaline and cortisol concentrations over time. Biol Psychiatry 2007;62(10):1095-102.
[85] Kassam-Adams N, Garcia-España JF, Fein JA, Winston FK. Heart rate and posttraumatic stress in injured children. Arch Gen Psychiatry 2005;62(3): 335-40.
[86] Pervanidou P, Chrousos G. Post-traumatic stress disorder in children and adolescents: from Sigmund's Freud's "trauma" to psychopathology and the (Dys)metabolic syndrome. Horm Metab Res 2007;39(6):413-9.
[87] Pervanidou P, Chrousos G. Post-traumatic stress disorder in children and adolescents: Neuroendocrine perspectives. Sci Signal 2012;5(245):6. doi. 10. 1126/ scisignal.2003327.
[88] Landolt MA, Vollrath M, Timm K, Gnehm HE, Sennhauser FH. Predicting posttraumatic stress symptoms in children after road traffic accidents. J Am Acad Child Adolesc Psychiatry 2005;44(12):1276-83.

[89] Winston FK, Kassam-Adams N, Vivarelli-O'Neill C, Ford J, Newman E, Baxt C, et al. Acute stress disorder symptoms in children and their parents after pediatric traffic injury. Pediatrics 2002;109(6):e90.
[90] Brand S, Otte D, Petri M, Decker S, Stübig T, Krettek C, et al. Incidence of posttraumatic stress disorder after traffic accidents in Germany. Int J Emerg Ment Health 2014;16(1):233-6.
[91] Noll-Hussong M, Herberger S, Grauer MT, Otti A, Gündel H. Aspects of post-traumatic stress disorder after a traffic accident. Versicherungsmedizin 2013;65(3):132-5. [German]
[92] Hours M, Chossegros L, Charnay P, Tardy H, Nhac-Vu HT, Boisson D, et al. Outcomes one year after a road accident: results from the ESPARR cohort. Accid Anal Prev 2013;50:92-102.
[93] Hours M, Khati I, Charnay P, Chossegros L, Tardy H, Tournier C, et al. One year after mild injury: Comparison of health status and quality of life between patients with whiplash versus other injuries. J Rheumatol 2014;41(3):528-38.
[94] Batailler P, Hours M, Maza M, Charnay P, Tardy H, Tournier C, et al. Health status recovery at one year in children injured in a road accident: A cohort study. Accid Anal Prev 2014;71:267-72.
[95] Tournier C, Charnay P, Tardy H, Chossegros L, Carnis L, Hours M. A few seconds to have an accident, a long time to recover: Consequences to road victims from the ESPARR cohort 2 years after the accicent. Accid Anal Prev 2014;72:422-32.
[96] Zink KA, McCain GC. Post-traumatic stress disorder in children and adolescents with motor vehicle-related injuries. J Spec Pediatr Nurs 2003;8(3):99-106.
[97] Kramer DN, Landolt MA. Early psychological intervention in accidentally injured children ages 2-16: A randomized controlled trial. Eur J Psychotraumatol 2014 Jun 27. doi: 10.3402/ejpt.v5.24402.
[98] Stallard P, Velleman R, Salter E, Howse I, Yule W, Taylor G. A randomized controlled trial to determine the effectiveness of an early psychological intervention with children involved in road traffic accidents. J Child Psychol Psychiatry 2006;47(2):127-34.
[99] Gillies D, Taylor F, Gray C, O'Brien L, D'Abrew N. Psychological therapies for the treatment of post-traumatic stress disorder in children and adolescents. Evid Based Child Health 2013;8(3):1004-116.
[100] Duzinski SV, Lawson KA, Maxson RT, Garcia NM, Calfa N, Metz K, et al. The association between positive screen for future persistent posttraumatic stress symptoms and injury incident variables in the pediatric trauma care setting. J Trauma Acute Care Surg 2012;72(6):1640-6.
[101] Suliman S, Stein DJ, Seedat S. Clinical and neuropsychological predictors of posttraumatic stress disorder. Medicine (Baltimore) 2014;93(22):e113. doi: 1097/MD.0000000000000113.
[102] Forman-Hoffman V, Knauer S, McKeenan J, Zolotor A, Bianco R, Lloyd S, et al. Child and adolescent exposure to trauma: comparative effectiveness of interventions addressing trauma other than maltreatment or family violence. Rockville (MD): Agency Healthcare Research and Quality, Report No: 13-EHC054-EF, 2013.

[103] Bisson JI, Roberts NP, Andrew M, Lewis C. Psychological therapies for chronic post-traumatic stress disorder (PTSD) in adults. Cochrane Database Syst Rev 2013;12:CD003388. doi: 10.1002/14651858.CD003388.pub.4
[104] Amos T, Stein DJ, Ipser JC. Pharmacologic interventions for preventing post-traumatic stress disorder (PTSD). Cochrane Database Syst Rev 2014;7:CD006239. doi: 10. 1002/14651858.CD006239.pub2.
[105] Parker AM, Sricharoenchai T, Raparla S, Schneck KW, Bienvenu OJ, Needham DM. Posttraumatic stress disorder in critical illness survivors: A metaanalysis. Crit Care Med 2015;43(5):1121-9.
[106] Meiser-Stedman R, Shepperd A, Glucksman E, Dalgleish T, Yule W, Smith P. Thought control strategies and rumination in youth with acute stress disorder and posttraumatic stress disorder following single-event trauma. J Child Adolesc Psychopharmacol 2014;24(1):47-51.
[107] Scheeringa MS, Salloum A, Arnberger RA, Weems CF, Amaya-Jackson L, Cohen JA. Feasibility and effectiveness of cognitive-behavior therapy for posttraumatic stress disorder in preschool children: two case reports. J Trauma Stress 2007;20(4):631-6.
[108] Ehlers A, Mahyou RA, Bryant B. Cognitive predictors of posttraumatic stress disorder in children: results from a prospective longitudinal study. Behav Res Ther 2003;41(1):1-10.
[109] Caffo E, Belaise C. Psychological aspects of traumatic injury in children and adolescents. Child Adolesc Psychiatr Clin North Am 2003;12(3):493-535.
[110] Salter E, Stallard P. Posttraumatic growth in child survivors of a road traffic accident. J Trauma Stress 2004;17(4):335-40.
[111] Di Gallo A. Injury to body and soul—psychiatric consequences of road traffic accidents in children and adolescents. Praxis (Bern 1994) 2005;94(12):467-70. [German]
[112] Schäfer I, Barkmann C, Riedesser P, Schulte-Markwort M. Posttraumatic syndromes in children and adolescents after road traffic accidents—a prospective cohort study. Psychopathology 2006;39(4):159-64.
[113] Bryant B, Mayou R, Wiggs L, Ehlers A, Stores G. Psychological consequences of road traffic accidents for children and their mothers. Psychol Med 2004;34(2):335-46.
[114] Wittman L, Zehnder D, Jenni OG, Landolt MA. Predictors of children's sleep onset and maintenance problems after road traffic accidents. Eur J Psychotraumatol 2012;3:8402. doi: 10.3402/ejpt.v3i0.8402.
[115] Stallard P, Smith E. Appraisals and cognitive coping styles associated with chronic post-traumatic symptoms in child road traffic accident survivors. J Child Psychol Psychiatry 2007;48(2):194-201.
[116] Williams JL, Rheingold AA, Knowlton AW, Saunders BE, Kilpatrick DG. Associations between motor vehicle crashes and mental health problems: Data from the National Survey of Adolescents-Replication. J Trauma Stress 2015;28(1):41-8.
[117] Cody MW, Beck JG. Physical injury, PTSD symtoms, and medication use: Examination in two trauma types. J Trauma Stress 2014;27(1):74-81.

[118] Landolt MA, Vollrath ME, Gnehm HE, Sennhauser FH. Post-traumatic stress impacts quality of life in children after road traffic accidents: prospective study. Aust NZ J Psychiatry 2009;43(8):746-53.
[119] Vermetten E, Olff M. Psychotraumatology in the Netherlands. Eur J Psychotraumatol 2013 May 2. doi: 10.3402/ejpt.v4i0.20832.
[120] Undavailli C, Das P, Dutt T, Bhoi S, Kashyap R. PTSD in post-road traffic accident patients requiring hospitalization in Indian subcontinent: A review on magnitude of the problem and management guidelines. J Emerg Trauma Shock 2014;7(4):327-31.
[121] Wu F, Meng WY, Hao CZ, Zhu LL, Chen DQ, Lin LY et al. Analysis of post-traumatic stress disorder in children with road traffic injury in Wenzhou, China. Traffic Inj Prev 2015 Nov 11. [Epub ahead of print]
[122] Merecz-Kot D, Waszkowska M, Wezyk A. Mental health status of drivers—Motor vehicle accidents perpetrators. Med Pr 2015;66(4):525-38. [Polish]
[123] Karsberg SH, Lasgaard M, Elkit A. Victimisation and PTSD in a Greenlandic youth sample. Int J Circumpolar Health 2012;71. doi: 10.3402/ijch.v71i0.18378.
[124] Mehta S, Ameratkunga SN. Prevalence of post-traumatic stress disorder among children and adolescents who survive road traffic accidents: A systematic review of international literature. J Paediatr Child Health 2012;48(10):876-85.
[125] Lilleston PS, Goldmann L, Verma RK, McCleary-Sills J. Understanding social norms and violence in childhood: theoretical underpinnings and strategy for intervention. Psychol Health Med 2017 Jan 9. doi: 10.1080/13548506.2016. 1271957. [Epub ahead of print].

Section one: The killing fields

In: Children and Youth
Editors: Donald E. Greydanus et al.
ISBN: 978-1-53611-102-6
© 2017 Nova Science Publishers, Inc.

Chapter 2

THE KILLING FIELDS ON THE ROADS: CAN WE PROTECT THE TEEN DRIVER?

Donald E Greydanus[*], *MD, DrHC(Athens)*
Department of Pediatric and Adolescent Medicine,
Western Michigan University Homer Stryker MD School of Medicine,
Kalamazoo, Michigan, US

This chapter considers the teenage driver and the high risk of injury as well as death that these young drivers represent for themselves and others because of automobile crashes in the United States and around the world. Research suggests that half a million teenagers will die as motor vehicle drivers or passengers in the 21st century, that 35 million adolescents will be injured as drivers in the 21st century, and untold millions of car passengers are at risk of death and/or injury when exposed to teenage drivers in this century. Reasons for the high prevalence of motor vehicle crashes with injuries and deaths are considered as well as measures that have been instituted over the past few decades to improve this situation. From a viewpoint of prospicience, it is hoped that more preventive measures along with more research will help to reverse this tragic trend in the 21st century.

---

[*] Correspondence: Donald E. Greydanus, MD, DrHC(Athens), Department of Pediatric and Adolescent Medicine, Western Michigan University Homer Stryker MD School of Medicine, Kalamazoo, MI 49008-1284, United States. E-mail: Donald.greydanus@med.wmich.edu.

INTRODUCTION

The United States (US) government's Centers for Disease Control and Prevention (CDC) notes that, in the United States, 71% of all deaths among persons aged 10–24 years in 2014 resulted from four causes: motor vehicle crashes (23%), other unintentional injuries (17%), homicide (14%), and suicide (17%) (1). The number one cause of death for American youths is the motor vehicle crash (cars, motorcycles, all-terrain vehicles, others) (2, 3). This young age group represents approximately 15% of the deaths from motor vehicle crashes in America and has been projected to conclude that half a million teenagers will die in the 21st century as drivers or passengers, 35 million will be injured as drivers, and untold millions are at risk of death and/or injury when exposed to teenage drivers in this century (4). This discussion considers these statistics, reviews underlying factors in these injuries as well as deaths, and provides some research-based solutions for some amelioration in the killings fields of the highways of America and around the world (4, 5).

OVERVIEW OF MOTOR VEHICLE CRASH DATA

The National Highway Traffic Safety Administration (NHTSA) collects information regarding motor vehicle crashes in the United States and though this data is an underestimation, it provides useful statistics for analysis of trends dealing mainly with car crashes (6, 7). For example, one motor vehicle crash-related death occurs in the context of 100 injuries not resulting in mortality. Teenage drivers who are 16-19 years of age have a four times increased rate of death versus the 25 to 69 year old driver; a nine-times increased in death is noted in the driver who is over 69 years of age. This is the tragedy inherited from the 20th century for the 21st century teenage driver, his/her passengers, involved parents, involved pedestrians, and for society in general (4, 5). Thus, it is fitting to briefly reflect on data from the period of transition of these two centuries and where such data is accumulated.

Late 20th century crash data

The United States Fatality Analysis Reporting System is a registry of motor vehicles deaths across the United States and a review of its 1991 to 1996 data revealed that 16,676 children under 16 years of age were killed as passengers, pedestrians, or bicyclists because of a motor vehicle crash; nearly 20% of these deaths involved crashes in which alcohol was involved (6).

Data from 1998 noted that 3,427 drivers who were between 15 and 20 years of age were killed in motor vehicle crashes (MVCs) while crash injures occurred to 348,000 (7). Statistics from 1998 recorded 7,975 drivers who were 15 to 20 years of age and involved in fatal motor vehicle crashes (MVCs)---- this represented 14% of all the recorded drivers in this situation with a total of 56,543 (4, 7). Drivers who were between 15 and 20 years of age represented 16% (1,801,000) of all drivers found in MVCs as reported by the police— 11,368,000 in total (4, 7). The projected cost of all these crashes was $31.8 billion in 1998 (7).

Early 21st century crash data

Unintentional injuries remain the leading cause of deaths among those 0-19 years of age in the United States and the leading cause for quantifying years of potential life lost (YPLL) in this age group between 2000 and 2009 was vehicle traffic-related injuries at 55% (8). Motor vehicle crashes are the number one cause of death for children ages 4 years and older (9). A review of the United States 2001-2010 Fatality Analysis Reporting System data notes that 2,344 children under age 15 years of age were killed in motor vehicle crashes that involved at least one driver who was alcohol-impaired; 65% were in the care of an alcohol-impaired driver (i.e., blood alcohol concentration of =0.08 g/dL (10).

In 2014, there were 1,717 young drivers 15 to 20 years old who died in motor vehicle crashes, an increase of 1 percent from 1,697 in 2013 (11). Additionally, an estimated 170,000 young drivers were injured in motor vehicle crashes in 2014, a decrease of 4 percent from 177,000 in 2013. Motor vehicle crashes are a leading cause of death for 15- to 20-year-olds, according to the 2014 data from the National Center for Health Statistics (11).

There were 214.1 million licensed drivers in the United States in 2014. Young drivers accounted for 5.5 percent (11.7 million) of the total, a 7-percent decrease from the 12.6 million young drivers in 2005 (11). The population for this age group decreased from 2005 to 2014 by 0.9 percent (11). Total fatalities in crashes with young drivers have decreased steadily over the 10-year period from 2005 to 2014, resulting in a 48-percent decrease in fatalities during that time (11). Fatalities among young drivers, the passengers of young drivers, and occupants of other vehicles all declined by approximately half (51%, 54%, and 44%, respectively). However, non-occupant fatalities in young-driver-related crashes decreased by only 28 percent during the same 10-year period (11).

In the United States, motor vehicle traffic crashes are the number one cause of unintentional injury-related deaths---leading to 33,687 deaths in 2010 (12). Motor vehicle crashes are the leading cause of death for those in the first three decades of life in the United States and the leading cause of death in those 10 to 24 years of age in the world (13). These crashes kill nearly 3,500 persons each day and injure or disable 50 million persons each year around the world (13). In 2013 there were 2,568 deaths of passenger vehicle drivers aged 16 to 19 years age involved in fatal vehicle crashes in the United States (12-14). This tragically high number of teenage driver deaths does reflect a 55% drop from 5,724 deaths in 2004 (14). Factors behind this decline are discussed later in this chapter (4, 5).

Pedestrian injuries and deaths

From 2001 to 2010, 47,392 pedestrians of all ages died from traffic crashes in the United States; this included 32,873 males and 14,519 females (12). Approximately 4,000 pedestrians of all ages die from crash-related injuries and about three fourths occur in urban areas. The pedestrian death rates increases with age (12).

Injuries can also occur to children from pedestrian injuries and studies note that pedestrian car accidents are one of the leading causes of death and injury in children (15). Tragically motor vehicle crashes (MVCs) are the leading cause of death for children 4 years and older (9). A 12 year-long study (1989-2001) of 501 children (0 to 16 years of age with average age of 7-9 years) concluded that lack of vehicle visibility and/or the child were major factors leading to the injury (15). The injuries were worse when the child was with other children versus being with adults or were alone as well as when speed at impact and no breaking attempts at impact occurred (15). Clinicians need to teach the public about issues involving cars and death in children that include child restraints (proper instillation and use), traveling in pickup trucks, children playing in and around motor vehicles, air bag exposure, and other issues (9).

Non-car crash death and injury

Death and injury can occur from crashes involving motorcycles, all-terrain vehicles (ATVs), bicycles, and other transportation crashes apart from or in connection with car crashes (4, 16-18). For example, all-terrain vehicle (ATV) deaths are noted in a study from 2007 to 2011 of the Fatality Analysis Reporting System (FARS) that revealed 1,701 ATV fatalities (17). The high death rate of crashes involving adolescents and young adults driving motorcycles remains of concern as well because of reckless driving behavior, lack of wearing helmets, use of drugs, and other factors (16-18).

In 2010 there were 3,951 reported deaths from motorcycle accidents in the United States in which 77% died at the accident scene, 10% died in the emergency department, and 13% died in the hospital; 69% of the deaths involved persons not wearing a helmet (16). During 2014, 225 motorcycle riders aged 15 to 20 years died in crashes that was a 4% reduction from 235 killed in 2013; 7,000 young drivers were injured in 2014---representing a 24% increase from approximately 6,000 in 2013 (11, 16, 18).

In 2009 there were 33,808 deaths from motor vehicle crashes in the United States that included 630 bicyclist deaths (19). In a study of the Fatality Analysis Reporting System (FARS) data from 1975 to 2012, there were 29,711 bicyclist deaths that included a decline in these deaths over this period---955 deaths in 1975 versus 717 in 2012. (19).

ANTECEDENTS TO TEENAGE MVC MORBIDITY AND MORTALITY

As noted, data derived by the Centers for Disease Control and Prevention as well as other researchers and organizations, motor vehicle crashes (MVCs) are the leading cause of death for children, adolescents, and young adults (1-15). A major factor in this carnage on the roads is the high injury and death rate for teenage drivers that not only kill or injury themselves, but many others caught in this violence. This discussion now considers some of the factors behind the potentially dangerous teen driver (see Table 1).

Table 1. Factors behind the dangerous teen driver

1. Adolescent development
2. Inexperience
3. Speeding
4. Distracted driving
5. The intoxicated driver (alcohol, cannabis, others)
6. Road rage
7. Medical issues
8. Vehicle technology issues (Seat belts, air brakes, seat bags, size)

Antecedents to increased accidents and deaths in teen drivers include adolescent development itself with inherent high risk-taking patterns, lack of driving experience, and patterns of unsafe (perilous) driving demeanor that includes driving under the influence of drugs (alcohol, cannabis, others) (20-26). Compared to some other countries, many American adolescents have ready access to a low-cost driver's license and a motor vehicle (26, 27).

The risk is the highest in the 16 to 17 years of age and this includes data showing that the crash rate per driven mile is nearly three times greater in 16 year old drivers versus 18 to 19 year old drivers (28, 29). These rates of MCAs and MCA-deaths are seen in males and two-thirds of adolescents killed in these accidents are males (28-31).

The modus operandi of teenage MCAs is that of a young driver involved in a single vehicle accident that involves high-speed roll-over crashes and run-off-the- road accidents (28-31). Single-car crashes are especially prone to death of the car occupant (s) and 21% of these crashes involve the young driver (4, 5, 30, 31). More persons are driving in daylight hours and thus, more MCAs occur during this time; however crashes that kill persons are more common at night. Daylight versus nighttime crashes can vary with age, usually lowering with increased age (4, 5, 26, 29). Some of these antecedents to potential teenage driving are now further considered.

ADOLESCENT DEVELOPMENT AND HIGH-RISK BEHAVIOR

Research over the past century has linked risky behaviors in many youth as they transition from childhood to adulthood (32). Young adolescents may not have developed the cognitive skills needed to avoid accidents while driving partially because they have not acquired safe driving skills which includes the capacity to acknowledge, pinpoint, analyze and then precisely evade driving impediments or imperilments faced by all divers over time—especially if unsafe driving behavior occurs (33-36). Developmental issues in adolescence include deficits for many in self-regulation, limited perception of safety issues, a need for thrill as well as adventure, driving before obtaining a license---all of which can result in unsafe driving for young teen drivers (37-42).

As compared to older drivers, young teens are often less skilled in keeping their motor vehicles at safe and legal speed limits. Partial cause of this dilemma includes the developing nature of adolescence---the skills of discernment, sophistication, and self-control are still being matured in the human transition phase called adolescence (24, 25, 43). These young drivers may not appreciate that their driving skills are limited and that they can play a direct role in causing accidents that injure and/or kill others as well as themselves.

Based on personality issues some teens are less safe drivers than others (43). US teens represent 40% of MVC deaths and such crashes by these novice drivers are characterized by recklessness, violating traffic laws, and single vehicle, rollover crashes (44). There are subgroups of novice drivers some of whom are more dangerous drivers than others and research in adolescent executive function as well as neuro-cognition (as measured in a driving stimulator and/or research questionnaires) may provide clues to safer driving by young drivers (45-47).

Society has long observed a dangerous sense of invulnerability found in many youth who drive---especially in males (34, 48-54). Indeed, the male adolescent (and sometimes the female as well!) may be a dangerous driver who does not honor or fear the potential dangers of heavy traffic, excessive speed, nighttime driving, tailgating, road rage, snow, ice, no-passing lanes, DWI (driving while intoxicated), distractions (phones, internet, turning one's head away while looking/talking), and other dangerous phenomena (31, 49, 55, 56).

Some drivers become caught up with the joy of driving a vehicle and/or the sense of power driving may provide (30, 31). Others may use driving to carry out struggles of suicidality with risk to themselves as well as potentially others (4, 31). More research is underway to identify potential links of high-risk driving with personality factors, attention-deficit/hyperactivity disorder, oppositional defiant disorder, and conduct disorder (57-60). Some of these issues are discussed later in this chapter.

Research also shows that being young is not always a negative trait with driving. For example, comparisons of young drivers and older drivers in terms of their visual response to headlight glare noted that the older driver had visual problems and not the younger ones (61). Also, a teen growing up in a stable family with a positive climate of teaching as well as supporting safe driving can blunt potentially reckless driving proclivities of adolescence (62). Research is needed on ways parents can influence improved driving skills in their young teen drivers (63).

OVERVIEW: DANGEROUS DRIVING HABITS OF YOUNG DRIVERS

Generation after generation of young drivers and teens in general have an increased propensity to drive in a dangerous manner---such as riding with a driving while intoxicated (DWI) driver, drive under the influence of drugs (alcohol, cannabis, others), perform illegal turns, drive through red lights, and others (28, 29, 64). Over half of MVCs involving teen drivers occur on weekends (i.e., Friday-Sunday) and over 40% occur between 9 PM and 6 AM (28, 29). Adolescents driving at night and especially after midnight sets up a high risk MCA situation combined with other high-risk factors discussed in this review (i.e., speeding, intoxication, multiple car passengers, others) (65). Some of these issues are now considered in more detail.

Inexperience

Motor vehicle driving involves a number of complex features that can cause problems for a young teen (or others) from any country who have no or minimal experience with driving performance (4, 5, 20, 66). The result of this inexperience is that poor choices may occur leading to accidents that research can probe further (21, 31, 52, 64). Motor vehicle crashes account for 30% of these deaths and are the number one cause of death in this age group (4, 5). An important cause of these deaths is the inexperience with driving skills that youth often possess along with increased risk taking behavior, dangerous driving patterns (such as excessive speed), and drug-impaired driving (i.e., alcohol, cannabis, others) (4, 5, 43, 44, 67).

The risk of motor vehicle crash for drivers of any age is the greatest during the first months of driving as independent drivers and the highest crash risk is among the youngest adolescent drivers during their initial independent driving period (14). This affects many adolescents in the United States as nearly 75% of those =16 years of age report they drove at least once during the 30 days of their YRBS (Youth Risk Behavior Surveillance) survey (14). This also places the passengers of these inexperienced drivers at great risk of injury and death as well.

It is a "catch-22" situation or as one research team described it with the term "young driver paradox" in which one needs to spend time driving to gain valuable experience and during that initial time the risk of accidents and poor decisions increases (68). It may take five years or so to become an "experienced" as well as safe driver and the individual who survives this time may become a safer, more efficient and reliable operator of a motor vehicle (30, 69).

This inexperience can lead to experimentation with a variety of unsafe driving behaviors influence by an inability to understand risks of unsafe driving. Teaching efforts aimed to the natural altruistic attitudes of many teens may be useful—i.e., safer driving will help others (70). Education should be targeted to deal with errors committed while under close supervision to correct such mistakes before they become habits (71). Teenage drivers should learn from programs that emphasize hazard anticipation training (72).

Teenagers (and all drivers) can be taught to improve their driving skills based on both their training but also as they gain experience (that may include errors made - i.e., learn from one's mistakes!). Education of experienced versus inexperienced drivers should be different as research suggests each group responds to different methods of training (73).

Speeding

One important part of dangerous driving behavior is speeding or going faster than the legal speed limits and/or operating a vehicle at a speed that is not safe for local driving conditions (4, 74). Studies note that over one-third (37% in one study) of male drivers (15 to 20 years of age) identified in fatal MVAs were speeding when the accident occurred (4, 5). The act of speeding is a major or primary factor in youth-related deadly MVCs and the underlying issue is that young drivers tend to drive faster than older, adult drivers (4). In a Colorado study of fatal motor vehicle crashes involving 16-year-old drivers that had 158 deaths in this age group from 1995 to 2001, speeding was one major factor contributing to these crashes (44).

Research concludes that young drivers embrace the potential for speeding and risky overtaking more than older drivers since youth tends to see the positive aspects of risky driving versus the potential negative consequences (4, 75). A number of factors can influence such dangerous behavior including identification with parents' driving habits, peer pressure to race and speed, limited media depictions of negative results of such driving, and as some have proposed---the automobile makers' advertisements promoting the speed of their cars (4, 5, 76).

Studies of youth suggest that as drivers they feel increased pressure from peers to speed as well as be involved in other risky driving behaviors that include tailgating, going through red lights and overtaking motor vehicles (77, 78). Racing can be part of popular movies as well. Research suggests that rid-light cameras may be useful for prevention of some drivers who go through red lights leading to crashes (79).

Peer influence is a major factor in young teen speeding and should be covered in any driver training that is provided (80). Further understanding of personal characteristics (attitudes), speeding to deal with personal depression, and concepts of reward sensitivity will also help understand reasons for speeding by young drivers and effective means to help them slow down (81). Young drivers must learn to avoid being pressured by peers to drive faster than the posted speed limits and faster than road conditions allow (74, 82).

Interviews of these younger drivers also reveals they simply do not conclude that speeding is a perilous act—in contrast to the older, adult driver (83). Education of these drivers should include such research concluding that on average speeding saves 26 seconds per day or 2 minutes per week in urban areas but leads to one death for every 24,450 hours saved and one injury for every 2,458 hour saved (84). Education should also identify those who say they speed to get a thrill and seek to carefully show that this "thrill" is not worth the risks in terms of injury and death to themselves and others (85). It is also vital to teach youth that pressure from peers to race and speed is a risky behavior that should be avoided for the safety of themselves and others (86).

Distracted driving

It is well-known that young teen drivers have a tendency to be involved in distracted driving (secondary task engagement) as influenced by listening to music, looking at cell phones or other internet devices, phone dialing, text messaging, and talking to (laughing with) other passengers (58, 66, 87, 88).

The 2015 Centers for Disease Control and Prevention (CDC) Youth Risk Behavior Surveillance (YRBS) reported that among the 61.3% who drive a car, 41.5% had texted or e-mailed while driving a car or other vehicle on at least one day during the 30 days prior to the survey (89).

Other issues of distraction which leads to diversion of attention needed for driving includes picking up an object, driver smoking, and distracting events outside of the car that can be combined with other interferences with driving skills such as sleep deprivation, alcohol use, and effects of psychotropic medications (90).

Unfortunately the driver becomes distracted with decrease in driving performance and increase in MVCs (87). The impact of this distraction is an increase in MVCs that kill an average of 8 persons per day in the United States and young drivers seem more incapacitated to safe driving while on the phone than older drivers (91, 92). Underlying mechanisms involve the dangers of a developing and sometimes faulty (inexperienced) executive function ability in many youth and young adults (93).

Complexities in the phenomenon of distracted driver behavior are made more difficult by research of varying quality in this important area (94). For example, it is challenging to scientifically measure the distractibility of social media technology while driving (95). Some research suggests that the general public seems to handle cell phone use without an increase in accidents and even teaches the driver how to pay attention to driving while phoning (96). Studies, however, do not usually support this optimistic view for teen drivers (91, 93, 97).

Research notes that 40% of drivers report talking on phones at least a few times per week and this tends to be reduced in states that ban such practices (98). Laws banning the use of driver cell phone use seem to have minimal effects on young teen drivers and may worsen the situation in some cases (99-101). Texting becomes an impulsive choice for some drivers and one difficult to stop (102).

Increased crash risks are noted for young drivers with passengers in the car, more for young (peer) passengers versus adult passengers (103). Though the effects of passengers on the teen driver are complex, driving simulator research suggests that it makes it more difficult for this young teen driver to safely operate a motor vehicle (103, 105). Having multiple passengers in a car leads to a less visual scanning range of male teen drivers and negative effects on the driver regarding real or perceived expectations as well as dangerous influences from the passenger (s) (106). Passengers may even seek to take over control of the vehicle or disrupt the internal milieu of the motor vehicle in other ways (107).

Correction or improvement of driver distraction has proven to be very challenging but teaching about safe rules of the road is imperative for any driver education course (91). A multi-pronged approach of education and legislation is needed to deal with risk factors of cellphone use and other social media while driving (108). Understanding of different personality traits involved in distracted driving behaviors would be helpful in devising effective strategies to stop this malignant behavior (109).

Use of digital games may be useful for young drivers (110). Teaching should include the principle that dangers from distracted driving rises as the duration of the distraction increases (111). Behavioral therapy strategies are needed to help teen drivers learn to avoid texting while driving and save lives (112). Different strategies are needed to deal with various mechanisms behind drivers using social interactive technology despite the risks (113).

Parent education to prevent their distracted driving may help their children avoid or reduce the tragedy of distracted driving behavior (DDB) (114, 115). Use of hands-free cell phones may be more beneficial than hand-held phones due to decreased cell phone visual-manual tasks that are needed (116). Reducing events involving driving with multiple passengers will lower crash risks for these younger drivers (117). Science of the 21st century reveals that the dangers to drivers, passengers, and pedestrians from distracted drivers due to texting and other distractions remains a serious problem and must be stopped—especially for the young teen driver (118, 119).

Though as noted, studies are mixed, some research suggests that carefully developed laws banning texting laws for drivers may have some positive impact especially on reducing deaths for young drivers (120). Use of universal texting bans along with delay of full driver's licensure may be beneficial in reducing this dangerous driving behavior (121, 122). The use of phone blocking software while driving is a potential effective tool in this war against distracted driver deaths (123). Improved vehicles (i.e., improved human-machine interface design; advanced driver assistance programs; other technologic advances) along with major public campaigns regarding the dilemma of distracted driver behavior may be useful as well (95, 124-127).

It remains a complex issue as drivers who say they support cell phone restrictions while driving also use this technology themselves (128). Passengers in cars with distracted drivers must be taught that they are in considerable danger of death for themselves in such tragic situations (129).

Health care personnel can be useful in teaching youth how to be good versus dangerous car passengers (130).

The intoxicated driver

Driving while intoxicated with alcohol, cannabis, and/or other drugs produces a very dangerous driver who causes tragic numbers of injury and death in themselves and others (4, 5). This discussion considers issues related to intoxication with alcohol and then cannabis.

The United States Youth Risk Behavior Surveillance Survey (YRBSS) is the largest public health survey system in the United States looking at various health behaviors in high school students. During the preceding 30 days of the survey, the 1997 US Youth Risk Behavior Survey noted that over one-third of high school students had ridden one or more times with a driver who had consumed alcohol (23). Also reported on this survey is that 17% (12% females, 21% males) indicated they drove a motor vehicle one or more times after alcohol consumption (23).

The 2015 YRBSS reported that 63.2% of high school students had had at least one alcohol drink on at least 1 day during their life and 32.8% had had at least one drink of alcohol on at least 1 day during the 30 days before the survey (called current alcohol use) (89). This survey also reported that 17.7% of students had five or more drinks of alcohol in a row (within a couple of hours) on at least 1 day during the 30 days before the survey. Among the 61.4% of students who drove a car or other vehicle during the 30 days before the survey, 7.8% had driven a car or other vehicle one or more times when they had been drinking alcohol (during the 30 days prior to the survey) (89). During the 30 days prior to the survey 20.0% of the students had ridden in a car or other vehicle one or more times with a driver who had been drinking alcohol (89).

Alcohol, driving, and teenagers/young adults

The prevalence of alcohol consumption and driving among high school students aged 16 to 19 years of age dropped from 22.3% in 1991 to 10.3% in 2011 (131). Though this represents a 54% drop, the high number of teenagers driving under the influence of alcohol remains alarming and represents a dangerous situation for these drivers, their passengers, other drivers, other passengers, pedestrians, and others in the way of these dangerous drivers. As noted, this situation is worsened by those driving under the influence of other drugs (i.e., cannabis, cocaine, others) with or without alcohol.

A motor vehicle crash or accident is identified as alcohol-related if either the driver or pedestrian has a blood alcohol concentration (BAC) of 0.01 g/dl or greater in the police report; a BAC of 0.10 g/dl or greater defines legal intoxication in most states (4, 7, 28). Motor vehicle crashes (MVCs) that are alcohol-related are typically single vehicle accidents that occur during late night hours (4, 7, 28). Driving under the influence of alcohol impairs the driver's ability and increases risk for MVCs and death. Driving under the influence of any psychoactive drug (alcohol, cannabis, others) is a serious public issue for contemporary society (132).

Males are more commonly involved in driving under the influence of alcohol and young male motor vehicle drivers involved in a fatal crash are at higher risk of consuming alcohol than young female drivers. Teenage drivers are at higher risk of a MVC under the influence of alcohol than older drivers regardless of the blood alcohol level (133).

Research has also shown that in the BAC range of 0.05 to 0.14, teenager drivers who are female are at nearly twice relative risk of being involved in a fatal MVC than males (134). Intoxicated drivers use seat belts less than non-intoxicated drivers and nearly three-quarters of young drivers of cars who had been drinking alcohol and were involved in fatal crashes were not wearing seat belt restraints (7).

Research also noted that over one-third of college students 18-24 years of age report they had ridden with a driver who had drank alcohol and over one-quarter of these students report they had driven a motor vehicle post-drinking alcohol during the 30 days period prior to this late 20th century survey (22, 23).

Riding with drivers under the influence of alcohol is critically important---nearly 20% of the deaths in alcohol-related MVAs are passengers (135). Since alcohol-related MVCs are a leading cause of mortality in teenagers, lives can be saved if we can reduce the number of persons who ride with drinking drivers. Indeed, it is important that we teach these passengers to avoid such behavior, that they should resist peer pressure to engage in such risky behavior, and that parents should be encouraged to teach their children to avoid this risky behavior as well (135). Children, adolescents, and young adults in the 21st century develop a positive attitude toward alcohol and cannabis that needs to be resisted by clinicians and society.

One risk factor for adolescents to be driving while intoxicated is early use of drugs in adolescence (136). We need to teach this young age group to avoid riding with a driver who is intoxicated with alcohol, cannabis, and/or any other intoxicating drugs; we also need to teach these young people that they should not be the persons driving while intoxicated. Part of the challenge in this intervention is that the intoxicated driver is typically a parent or other household adult of the passenger or passengers (137). Risky driving behaviors of adults are very dangerous as modeling behaviors for teen and young adult drivers.

A vigorous campaign is needed to teach adolescents and others to be careful to get into a car with risky drivers, as many factors enter into their potential death in a car crash. These factors include speeding, an intoxicated driver, mobile phones, no seat belt use, late-night driving, absence of a valid driver's license, and/or having multiple car passengers who are typically fellow teenagers (66, 138). Death rates rise as more of these factors are present.

Other research concludes that Caucasian males from western or northern states in the United States are at the highest risk of drinking and driving, especially those living in rural areas (139). Factors associated with drinking and driving activity include the presence of teenagers having a history of truancy and drug abuse while there is also positive associations with increasing miles driven per week and the number of evenings out; protective factors include good academic achievement and being classified as "religious" (139).

Further data of alcohol-fueled death and destruction

In 1998 the United States Department of Transportation. National Highway Traffic Safety Administration concluded that approximately 30% of Americans would be involved in an alcohol –related automobile vehicle accident at some point in their lives (7, 140). Such accidents were seen in 57% of motor vehicle deaths and 21% of drivers aged 15-20 years of age who were killed in MVCs were legally intoxicated (7, 140).

A national study in the United States of the Fatality Analysis Reporting System between 1991 and 1996 identified 16,676 children younger than 16 years of age killed in a MVC either as passengers, pediatricians, or bicyclists (6). Drivers who were younger than the legal drinking age of 21 who consumed alcohol were identified in 30.3% of these pediatric deaths (6).

A descriptive study of 2001-2010 Fatality Analysis Reporting System data (United States) for child passengers under 15 years of age reported that 2,344 children were killed; 65% were in the car of an alcohol-impaired driver (10). One-third of these impaired drivers did not have a valid drivers' license and 61% of the dead children were not restrained in the car at the time of the crash (10). Research suggests that about 20% of children killed as motor vehicle passengers in the U.S. were in a vehicle with a driver who was impaired by alcohol who usually was the child's driver (10). Some states (i.e., California, Texas, South Dakota, New Mexico) has more impaired drivers than others based on local laws seeking to protect children and others (10).

In 2015 the Centers for Disease Control and Prevention reported on 2002-2014 data from the Substance Abuse and Mental Health Services Administration (SAMHSA) National Survey on Drug Use and Health (NSDUH) (132). This U.S. Centers for Disease Control and Prevention (CDC) publication concluded that the reported prevalence of driving under the influence of alcohol alone was greater than that of cannabis alone or the combination of cannabis with alcohol. The reported prevalence of driving under the influence of alcohol for those aged 16-20 years dropped from 16.2% in 2002 to 6.6% in 2014. The reported prevalence of driving under the influence of alcohol for those 21 to 25 years of age also dropped from 29.1% in 2002 to 18.1% in 2014 (132).

The reported prevalence of driving under the influence of alcohol and cannabis for those 16 to 20 years of age dropped from 2.3% in 2002 to 1.4% in 2014; this reported prevalence (driving under the influence of alcohol and cannabis) dropped for 21 to 25 year olds from 3.1% in 2002 to 1.9% in 2014. The reported prevalence of driving under the influence of alcohol increased from 1.5% for 15 year olds in 2014 to 18.1% for 21 year old drivers (132).

Another research group concluded that teenage students who drink and drive report use of cannabis, experiences with other alcohol using drivers as well as direct intentions to drive after drinking; they also note that their impaired driving gets them into conflicts with friends, school individuals, and parents (141). These youth report felling pressure from peers to drink and drive and they were thus more likely to be do this action in contrast those who could resist such peer pressure; they also were more tolerant of being in a car with an alcohol-impaired driver if these youth concluded they could safely drink and drive. Youth who report lack of self confidence in staying away from such behavior were more likely to engage in such risky behavior as drinking and driving.

Reasons for such dangerous driving behavior in teenage drivers resulting in high risk for fatal crashes remain under study but a number of theories have arisen. Such hypotheses include late 20th century speculation that these young drivers have a special "sensitivity" to alcohol and alcohol impairs driving skills to a greater extent in these young drivers versus older drivers; the complex effects of alcohol in youth may lead to an increased tendency to engage in such actions without fear of negative consequences (142-144).

Cannabis

An early reflection on the dangers of cannabis and driving can be seen in an article in 1976 (145). Research notes that cannabis-intoxicated drivers continues to be a serious issue leading to MVCs and partially fueling this trend is 21st century society's growing tolerance and acceptance of cannabis (67, 146, 147). The literature on the deadly combination of cannabis and driving with or without alcohol or other drugs continues to accumulate as more teenagers and adults die from this deadly combination (148-160).

The 2015 YRBSS reported that during the 30 days prior to the survey, 21.7% had used marijuana, while 38.6% of these students had used this drug one or more times in their life (89). As noted, many teenagers and young adults (including college students) operate a motor vehicle under the influence of cannabis which can lead to driving impairments and subsequent risks for accidents and death (67, 148, 157-162).

A published report by the U.S. Department of Transportation (DOT) notes that the prevalence of driving on weekend nights under the influence of cannabis for drivers = 16 years increased by 48% from 2007 to 2013-2014; it was 8.6% in 2007 and 12.6% in the 2013-2014 survey (163). The presence of cannabis was determined by biochemical assays in this DOT report (163).

Road rage

Road rage is another reason for dangerous driving behavior in a number of drivers but especially young male drivers, those driving in busy urban areas, and those with high powered cars where speeding may be hindered by urban congestion (164). Road rage driving increases the risks for MVCs that can be deadly to many around the world (165-169). Current research suggests that drivers who have suffered a traumatic brain injury are at increased risk for aggressive driving that can result in MVCs (170).

Driving a motor vehicle under the influence of alcohol, cannabis, and/or other drugs increases road rage risks (171-173). Drivers involved in road rage incidents typically display anger in other arenas of their lives that can include a high number of police-issued citations, bar fights, wall punching when angry, running other drivers off the road, and various psychiatric co-morbidity (including borderline personality disorder and attention-deficit/hyperactivity [ADHD]) (172, 174-176).

On psychological testing some young drivers demonstrate a tendency for driving anger and angry hostility (169, 177). Drivers who report anger while driving can also report anger in non-driving situations (178). A significant predictor of traffic fatality rate in a community is its homicide rate and such acts are part of an aggressive milieu that includes road rage driving (179). The sociologic theory of "homogamy" has been applied to being victims of it themselves (180).

Management of road rage is difficult and is related to dealing with persons having an aggressive view of living. Part of the difficulty in establish beneficial management principles for road rage is the inconsistency found in researchers and clinicians regarding even the definition of road rage (181). Merely warning such drivers about their behavior is often ineffective--- such as telling them that road congestion is ahead and they should avoid being frustrated by such traffic conditions (182). However, education is still needed to teach drivers of road rage events to avoid being sensitized by various events that increase their anger that erupts later into tragic road rage incidents (183).

Parents should be taught that if they have risky driving behavior (including aggressive driving), this can be associated with road rage events in their sons; this trait is particularly seen in a father-son road rage association (184). Persons in treatment for drug dependence should be clearly taught about the association between substance use and road rage behavior (173). Those with attention-deficit/hyperactivity disorder (ADHD) should receive instruction in driver's training about the potential link between ADHD and aggressive driving (176).

Experts suggest a multi-tiered approach to road rage in society that involves judicial punishment for such acts, court-appointed programs for these transgressors, motor vehicle designs to restrict cars from being used in road rage, education of the public to the problem of road rage, and other prevention efforts that include less traffic congestion, increased access to public transportation, and other means to reduce stress in humans (185).

Research suggests different subtypes of drivers with road rage based on the state-trait theory and the need for different approaches for different personality sub-types (186, 187). Persons with a history of traumatic brain injury (TBI) should be educated about the association of TBI with aggressive driving (170). Those with anger should be taught to avoid taking their anger out on others including cyclists who are in danger from aggressive motor vehicle drivers (188).

MEDICAL ISSUES OF YOUNG DRIVERS

Medical issues of young and all drivers can present potential problems for drivers, passengers, pedestrians, governments, and society in general. These issues involve a wide variety of medical disorders including neurodevelopmental and medical conditions. For example, if the car driver has epilepsy, unsafe driving practices may occur if this condition is not well-controlled. Laws regarding when persons with epilepsy can drive vary from state to state and country to country though all laws require a specific period of time without seizures as defined in a specific state or country law (189). The driver with unstable seizure disorder presents a danger to society if s/he disobeys local laws in this regard (190)

Another medical disorder that may present problems for drivers and society is the driver with poorly controlled diabetes mellitus that can lead to accidents if hypoglycemia or hyperglycemia occurs while driving (191). In one study of adolescent drivers with type 1 diabetes mellitus, over half of their parents worried about this issue and some of these parents noted their teen drivers had been in a motor vehicle accident (MVA) or had been stopped by police because of abnormal blood sugars in these teen drivers (191). Such issues are poorly studied and require more research in the 21st century.

A drowsy driver, young or older, suffering from a sleep debt is a dangerous driver who has an increased risk for deadly MVCs; perhaps 15% to 33% of fatal crashes involve a sleepy driver (192-195). There are many reasons for such drowsiness besides poorly controlled medical disorders. As children progress from childhood to adolescence, many develop a change in their circadian rhythms that lead to later bedtimes that can induce sleepiness when required early rising for school cuts into critical needs for sleep (196, 197). School regions that have allowed later school start times have seen a decreased risk for teen driver-induced MVAs (198, 199). Also, teenagers may have a variety of sleep disorders, such as sleep apnea, that may not be diagnosed but place the driver at increased risk for MVAs (196, 197, 200-202).

Also of concern involves the many drivers with neurodevelopmental disorders such as autism spectrum disorder (ASD) and attention-deficit/hyperactivity disorder (ADHD) (203). For example, teenagers with high-function ASD can learn to drive but they need comprehensive driving education (i.e., improving working memory) as well as evaluation of driving performance (i.e., using a driving simulator) to certify that a specific person with ASD is fit to drive and possesses critical executive functions as well as basic motor skills (204-207).

ADHD has received specific attention by researchers with regard to driving skills that may be impaired by such ADHD traits as inattention and impulsivity that may require medication to improve (208). Young drivers with ADHD seem to have increased risk for MVAs due to these issues that includes an overestimation of ability, increased risk taking, and increased problems with distraction (209-211). Special driving education programs and use of medication (i.e., stimulants) can be an important aspect of encouraging safer driving by young teen drivers with ADHD (208, 212).

AUTOMOBILE TECHNOLOGY: SEAT BELTS

Another aspect of risky driving habits is the failure to wear seat belts and this behavior can be measured in various ways such as self-report studies that in adults can correlate with observed measures in adult drivers (213). Safety belts for cars have been standard aspects of cars since 1968 in the United States and lap shoulder belts were added in the 1970s that can lower death for those in the car's front seats by 50% (214). Use of seat belts can save lives as noted by a 2000 to 2014 study of teen driving deaths and injuries in the State of Alabama (215).

Seat belt use significantly reduces the risk of traumatic brain injury and other injuries to the head, face, and neck (216). It can increase thoracic to coccyx injury but the severity of this injury (i.e., fracture) is less with use versus non-use of seat belts (216). Medical costs of injuries in a MVA are much lower with use of seat belts versus non-use (216). Increased safety is true for drivers of all ages and all motor vehicles if seat belts are regularly used---even long-haul truck drivers (217).

Research consistently records low seat-belt use by teenagers that contributes to MVAs and high teenage death rates (218). One study comparing teenage and adult drivers' use of seatbelts reported that novice drivers within one year of their license were the most likely of drivers to use seatbelts—the second group with the highest seat belt use were older drivers followed by middle-aged drivers and then young drivers (219). A subgroup of teen drivers with low seat belt use (as well as driving under the influence of alcohol and/other drugs) is the unlicensed teenage driver (220). In this national study, 4.2% of 9th to 11th graders reported they drove at least 1 hour/week without a license (220).

Failure to use seat belts while driving has been seen in over 20% of youth—23.2% in one study of high-school males and 14.5% of high-school females who were passengers in a motor vehicle (2). The 2015 CDC YRBSS (Youth Risk Behavior Surveillance Survey) reported that 6.1% of high school students rarely or never wore a seat belt when riding in a car driven by someone else (89). In a study of college students, 12.3% of the males and 6.6% of the females rarely or never used seat belts (22). In a Colorado study of fatal motor vehicle crashes involving 16-year-old drivers using the US Fatality Analysis Reporting System (FARS), seatbelt nonuse was seen in 48% of these novice drivers (44).

Though seat belt use can save lives, it has not been accepted by some drivers and passengers. Theorized reasons for limited seat belt by youth include modeling influence of peers, limited concerns with motor vehicle crashes, desire for comfort unhindered by seat belts, acceptance of myths stating seat belts are useless, and enjoyment of not complying with laws or requirements (221). Peer approval of seat belt use seems to be more influential or important for many teens than acquiescing to laws about seat belt use.

Laws that mandate seat belt use are helpful in protecting the public, as for example increasing use of seat belts from 11% in 1980 to over 75% in 1995 (214). This leads to less deaths and less non-fatal injuries and should be encouraged for all persons in a car. Mandatory seat belt use is more effective if it is part of a community's primary enforcement law in which police are able to stop a driver for not wearing a seat belt. This is in contrast to the less effective secondary enforcement law in which the police can stop and ticket a driver if other issues are being violated (214).

AUTOMOBILE TECHNOLOGY: AIRBAGS, CHILD CAR SEATS, AND ANTILOCK BRAKES

Automatic airbags can lower risks of death in a crash though it can pose problems for small children. Child car seats are useful to improve the safety of children in motor vehicles but they may be used incorrectly and concern has been raised with injuries and death in children caused by air bags (222). Antilock brakes are another safety feature provided by the automobile industry though it may lead to accidents as well, especially for new drivers not used to such devices (223-225).

AUTOMOBILE TECHNOLOGY: VEHICLE SIZE

Improvements in car technology for safety is important for drivers and passengers in the 21st century as well as reduction in MVC-induced health care costs (226). A motor vehicle that has a large size and weight is much safer to drive than one that is smaller and lighter. A vehicle's "crash-worthiness" is an important concept for drivers and passengers to comprehend—especially novice drivers and the involved families who must learn that the young driver and passengers are safer in a larger, heavier car with everyone in seat belts (224).

Research notes that if a MVC occurs between two vehicles with one car having a two-times the mass difference versus the other car, the lighter car driver has a 12 times greater risk of being killed than the heavier car driver (223, 227). In general, a driver of a smaller car has a two-three times risk of dying in the crash versus the driver of the heavier car (225).

Vehicle sizes, as well as other features such as seat belts, are good safety components for cars that involve various degrees of choice and selection. Another major safety feature is electronic stability control (ESC) that reduces the risks of being in a serious MVC (228). Current style air bags can save lives for child passengers in the car's right front during frontal collisions (229).

OTHER TECHNOLOGY: HELMETS

Other safety features are important as for example the reduction in death for motorcycle drivers and bicycle riders who regularly wear helmets (230, 231).

The best way to provide effective motorcycle rider training to prevent MVCs is unclear at this time (232). Improved motorcycle and bicycle technology has also saved lives as well. This discussion now turns to consideration of strategies of dealing with high risk teen driver behavior.

Table 2. Preventive measures of the last quarter of the 20th century

Drivers Education Program
Graduated Licensing System (GLS)
Zero tolerance laws for alcohol
Minimum drinking age laws
Designated driver concept
Ignition lock devices
Administrative per se laws
Random drug (alcohol) screening
Mandatory safety belt use
Larger vehicles
Airbags

STRATEGIES FOR DEALING WITH HIGH RISK TEEN DRIVING BEHAVIOR

A number of strategies have been considered and even implemented over the past decade in attempts to mitigate the high morbidity and mortality seen with young, inexperienced, and sometimes reckless young adolescent drivers of motor vehicles (see Table 2). What has not worked is the traditional education of young drivers of the 20th century. Some benefit has been seen with a graduated licensing system (GLS), increasing the legal age for alcohol consumption to age 21 years, and strict enforcement of strengthened drunk driving legislation (224).

Driver education

An initial program to teach drivers how to drive was developed in 1916 and it was used for the next several decades though its effectiveness was not measured (28). The United States used its Federal Department of

Transportation to have driver education programs for high school students become standard by the 1970s though fewer students have received such pedagogy for the past quarter of a century (233). As the 20th century came to a close, less than 25% of high school students receive formal drivers' education in some areas (4).

An initial (1976) thorough evaluation of drivers' education effectiveness was performed in the DeKalb County, Georgia public school system and concluded that minimal effectiveness in lowering risky teenage driving resulted from such attempts (233). The 1999 conclusion by the Insurance Institute for Highway Safety was that the education allowed an easy way for the learner to get through the course but provided minimal attention to "supervised practice and training" (4, 26).

Simple testing of basic driver skills and/or knowledge did not help reduce MVCs nor reduce the dangers of the initial teen male driver (4, 140, 234, 235). Such inadequate training may have worsened the situation by allowing a teen driver with an innate sense of invulnerability to increase this dangerous feeling of doing anything without negative consequences behind the wheel. The use of driver simulator training per se has not been proven to reduce teenage MVCs and more research is needed to maximize potential benefit from this technology (236).

A variety of driver education programs have been tried over the past decades and continue to be refined. Involving teenagers in the development of effective training programs is recommended as well as looking at how to build resilience into teenage driving programs (237, 238). Involving parents in driver education programs is also an important potential step in helping teenagers become safer drivers (239-242). Parents can model proper driver behavior and help limit novice teen driving (240).

Looking at drivers' innate patterns and driving styles as well as driver's personality may be helpful in correcting bad habits that may increase a specific driver's risk of accidents (243, 244). An example is research looking at those who drive with various jerks or "jerky driving" (245). This pattern of driving leads to increased accidents and if found, should be corrected.

Research then focused on training novice drivers as there was no evidence that post-license driver education prevented MVCs (246). It was of concern at the turn of the 20th century that studies concluded driver education among teenagers was not effective in preventing MVAs (247). Other research looked at hazards of driving on rural roads versus urban roads and this can be incorporated into driver training programs depending on where the young driver lives (248).

Graduated Driver Licensing System (GDLS)

A number of suggestions have been made already in this discussion to improve driver education in youth. One of the best innovations in driver education over the past decades has been the Graduated Driving Licensing System (GDLS), also called GLS (Graduated Licensing System) which has implemented an extended learner permit period for novice teen drivers and developed restrictions (i.e., car passengers, night driving). The GDLS was developed to help new and typically young teen drivers slowly integrate into real-life traffic conditions so they can become safer drivers provided with helpful skills, knowledge, and early experience (140, 249).

By the mid-1990s a few states had begun an early GLS laws and between 1996 and 2006 all states had elements of this system that included 2 months or longer as a driver learner, certain hours of supervised driver practice, and other GLS elements (250). All states now have some form of a GLS for its teenager drivers but more progress and universal tight legislation is needed to save more teenage lives. Unfortunately minimal progress has been made in many states over the past decade or more (250).

The hope is that uniform GLS training will provide earlier experience leading to more maturity and judgement behind the wheel of a vehicle (251). Such a program requires gradual driving experience over an extended time and involves increased supervised driving experience in contrast to previous driver education programs. There is training during daytime and nighttime, training in basic as well as advanced driving skills, and pressure placed on the learner to have time without any MVAs before obtaining the coveted, full driver licensure (7, 52, 140, 249).

GLS training that restricts nighttime driving is an important aspect of training to study for it reduces nighttime teen crashes (252-255). GLS also reduces miles (kilometers) driven and the number of driving trips by 16 and 17 year old novice drivers (256). Another positive benefit of graduated driver licensing laws is that it can teach as well as order social norms and expectations for adolescents and their risky driving behaviors (257).

Some research concludes that a graduated licensing system emphasizes the importance of a proper attitude toward driving that is a critical factor in promoting safety (4, 7, 50). Successful GLS broadens the education process for the young learner because it reduces exposure to risks of driving while improving driving proficiency and reduces fatal and non-fatal crashes by young, novice teen drivers (4, 258-260).

The period needed from the first initial driver's permit to full licensure is lengthened and includes initial minimal nighttime driving and more supervision by parents (4, 7). How long should the learner's permit be extended---research suggests at least 6 months (259). If driving mistakes occur early, it allows their correction before full licensure occurs and motivates the young driver to acquire safe driving skills (Table 2). How effective is this program in saving lives of 16 and 17 year old drivers---perhaps an 8 to 14% reduction in deaths of these drivers will be seen (261).

The exact impact on lives saved remains to be determined by further research as well as which components of GLS are the most effective (262, 263). Strong components of these programs include delayed licensing and night driving restrictions which saves young teen drivers' lives (264, 265). Some research shows that the supervised driving of young drivers in the GLS may be improved to save more lives (266).

GLS programs only deal with new drivers under 18 years of age in nearly all states and thus, those who apply for a driver's license after age 18 years are not in the GLS program (267). Extending the GLS program beyond age 17 may help to reduce MVC rates in older teenagers (268). Extending GLS training to all novice drivers will benefit those who do not begin driving until after their 18th birthday due to socioeconomic or other driving delaying factors (269, 270).

Support for the GLS has been seen in various areas including in legal circles, medical circles, parents, school personnel and the insurance industry (7, 50, 271). The NHTSA (4, 7, 50) has recommended a two stage program in which the initial education deals with skills needed during the early phase of driver education which can result in a restricted license. In the second phase steps are taken to improve skills of decision-making to lower risks of driving (4, 7).

Studies note that these programs and night-time curfews reduce young driver-related MVCs---such crashes lead to deaths as well as injuries to the teen driver and others (50, 249). Delayed licensing for teen drivers can save lives as noted by a 2000 to 2014 study of teen driving deaths and injuries in the State of Alabama (272). GLS delays teenage driving but does not result in increased deaths for passengers, pedestrians, bicyclists, or bus riders as a result (273).

Based on research from the Naturalistic Teenage Driving Study, it was concluded that GLS should also focus on improving teenage kinematic risky driving behavior to reduce crashes in these vulnerable drivers (274). Kinematic risky driving refers to the rate of increased gravitational-force events per 100 miles based on data received via accelerometers and global positional systems (274).

More research is needed to improve training for drivers in this post-Graduated Driver Licensing era as some research describe a sharp increase in crash risk for drivers who transition from intermediate to full licensure due to various factors---such as potential change in driving time, dangerous driving behaviors, and others as identified in this discussion (275). As noted earlier, it takes several years to develop driving skills to be able to be a safe driver on the dangerous, killing fields (roads) of America (4). Laws that increase the time unsupervised drivers must spend in supervision before being allowed to drive alone will save injuries and lives (276).

Alcohol (and other drug) related measures

Intense societal approaches are important to lower the high prevalence of driving while intoxicated (DWI) and riding with intoxicated drivers (RWI) (277, 278). As noted DWI also involves other aspects of risky driving such as speeding, being distracted, tailgating, and others in which the driver's attention becomes divided leading to MVCs (278, 279). A trend in the 21st century is that driving while intoxicated also means driving under the negative influence of prescription drugs in addition to cannabis and even multiple drugs (280, 281).

The most beneficial programs that have been utilized to lower teenage drivers' MVCs are minimum driving age laws and drunk driving laws (license suspension laws as well as zero tolerance laws) (4, 7, 139). For example, research has concluded that zero tolerance for drivers having any detectable alcohol or a blood alcohol concentration (BAC) with a maximum of 0.2g/dl in drivers under 21 years of age leads to lower nighttime fatal MVCs (single vehicle) in teenagers; this trend increases with lower BAC (4, 7).

The application of zero tolerance for teenage drivers lowers fatal single vehicle accidents (the type most common in youth) by 20%. In terms of drivers involved in fatal MVCs and drivers who were killed between 1988 and 1998, there was a 49% lowering of drivers aged 15 to 20 who were intoxicated (4, 7).

Indeed, the data is powerful in indicating the benefit of restricted BAC laws (282). All 50 states and the District of Columbia in the United States have a minimal drinking law of 21 years of age and such laws lower traffic fatalities by 13% in which drivers were 18 to 20 years of age with untold thousands of lives saved (4, 7, 139). Many states have a 0.08 g/dl as the legal intoxication limit and zero tolerance for drivers under age 21 are seen in all 50 states and the District of Columbia. It is against the law for drivers to operate a motor vehicle if they are under 21 years of age and have a BAC level of 0.02 g/dl or more.

As already noted, the reported prevalence of driving under the influence of alcohol for those aged 16-20 years dropped from 16.2% in 2002 to 6.6% in 2014. The reported prevalence of driving under the influence of alcohol for those 21 to 25 years of age also dropped from 29.1% in 2002 to 18.1% in 2014 (132).

The reported prevalence of driving under the influence of alcohol and cannabis for those 16 to 20 years of age dropped from 2.3% in 2002 to 1.4% in 2014; this reported prevalence (driving under the influence of alcohol and cannabis) dropped for 21 to 25 year olds from 3.1% in 2002 to 1.9% in 2014. The reported prevalence of driving under the influence of cannabis alone was the influence of alcohol that increased from 1.5% for 15 year olds in 2014 to 18.1% for 21 year old drivers (132).

Getting alcohol and other drug impaired drivers (i.e., with cannabis, cocaine, others) off the road will also save thousands of car passengers and pediatricians killed by these drivers; many of those killed are children (10). Male and female adolescents must be taught more effectively to avoid drinking and driving. Though males are often targeted as being intoxicated drivers, research shows that female adolescents often get involved in various dangerous driving behaviors that include driving under the influence of alcohol and other drugs (283). Some countries are encouraging use of public transportation and running campaigns that "Drinking and Driving Do not Mix"—encourage those who drink and drive to not drive (i.e., use public transportation especially at night) (284).

We can also save many lives by teaching potential car passengers to avoid riding in a car with a drinking driver and a model predicting such behavior has been studied (135). This includes teaching children to avoid being in a car with such drivers whether they are using alcohol, cannabis, or other drugs (136). We need to improve the lack of effective communication between adults and adolescents about the dangers teenagers and others being with alcohol impaired drivers (285). The compounded tragedy of deaths from alcohol/drug-related MVCs is that along with deaths of teenagers and adults is the deaths of children who are passengers; one in 5 child passenger deaths in the U.S. involves an alcohol-impaired driver (10). The US NHTSA estimates that

277,742 persons were saved from 2005 to 2014 by minimum drinking age laws (11).

Designated driver concept

Research also concludes that the concept of the designated driver can prevent teenage accidents and deaths; it is supported by the NHTSA (282, 286). Some suggest this policy will stimulate motor vehicle passengers to consume extra alcohol since they will feel "protected" by having a sober driver (286). A study of students in American colleges who were alcohol drinkers reported that over one-third had been a designated driver; though 40% had a history of binge drinking, none did when serving as a designated driver (286). Some, however, will binge drink when having a driver who had not been drinking prior to operating the motor vehicle (286).

Ignition interlock devices

Ignition interlock devices have been used to prevent intoxicated drivers from operating a vehicle (287). The driver who wishes to drive a car with such a device must provide a breath sample and if the level is above a specified level, the ignition remains locked. Many states and local districts have laws that utilize this method for those involved with DWI recidivism. Some studies note this as an effective tool for many to prevent drunk driving (287).

Administrative per se laws

In the "administrative per se" law (s) the concept is that a person's legal right to drive a motor vehicle can be suspended as a punishment if found driving under the influence of alcohol and this suspension does not depend on having the addition of having a statutory offense or if the person is found guilty (or innocent) of other offenses (288). In this legal argument the fact of failing a BAC test can lead to revoking one's driver's license. In some research such a concept has been found beneficial in reducing alcohol-related MVCs in drivers with a history of such offenses (288). Not all research agrees with this conclusion and more studies are needed in this regard (288).

Laws seeking to influence safe driving can have beneficial effects on some drivers of all ages. For example, studies on the benefit of using speed cameras to slow drivers down show that most drivers will lower their speed when they see these devices; the impact of young drivers remains unclear (289-292). Education about the benefits of seat belts along with law enforcement can improve drivers' as well as car passengers' use of seat belts (293). Education strategy that promote seat belt education as well as social pressure to use seat belts can increase their use as well in adolescents (294).

If drivers use seat belts, their front seat passengers are more likely to use seat belts as well (295). A national telephone survey of 1,218 persons 18 years of age and older noted that many (especially if they always use seat belts) would encourage their passengers to use them and would accept belt reminders for passengers, particularly children in the back; these drivers would accept an alert if children in the back became unbuckled (296). Education about use of seat belt in high school programs have shown improvement in seat belt use by teenage drivers (218).

Random screening programs

Such programs are based on the belief that some drivers will be deterred from drinking and driving if they believed they may be caught and punished. This program based on issues of deterrence and enforcement have received mixed reviews in research. Some research notes it is helpful in reducing alcohol-related MVCs for a short time while others note a more prolonged effect (297).

Effectiveness is seen if there are effective laws behind it, that the punishment for getting caught is clear as well as meaningful, and the public is educated to the presence of such laws in their communities (297). Communities with increased police patrols can reduce alcohol-impaired driving though more research is needed to maximize its efficacy (298). Interventions on the alcohol server setting have not proven beneficial in reducing alcohol intoxication—though research is limited in this area (298).

Vehicle-related measures

Protection of drivers, passengers, and pedestrians is an important measure in reducing injury and MVC sequelae such as PTSD. Unfortunately parents and teen drivers may use factors other than car size/weight in selecting a car---

using such features, for example, as gas mileage, and ignoring such safety features as side airbags or electronic stability control (225, 300). Many issues need to be considered in selecting cars for young drivers. For example, cars that are too quiet can present danger for drivers and pedestrians since these cars may be difficult to be heard (301).

Also, confusing the issue of car safety is research noting that some small cars are as "safe" as larger cars in some frontal collisions (302). However, parents and society must understand that teen drivers in unsafe cars (i.e., involving factors as size, type, and age) leads to increased death as well as injuries for these young drivers and their passengers (227, 303, 304). Constant education of the public to factors that provide protection in MVCs and those that do not remain important in the 21st century---especially targeted to vulnerable drivers such as teen drivers and their parents (305, 306).

CONCLUSION

In this consideration on the teenage driver, various issues have been considered including statistics related to morbidity and mortality for teen drivers, passengers, and pedestrians in the 20th and 21st centuries. Roadways should be considered killing fields for thousands of human beings involved in motor vehicle crashes (MVCs) (4, 5). Injuries and deaths can occur with any vehicle including automobiles, trucks, all-terrain motor vehicles, motorcycles, bicycles, and others. Also considered are factors that influence such death and injuries such as adolescent development, inexperience, speeding, distracted driving, the intoxicated driver (alcohol, cannabis, other drugs), road rage, medical issues, and vehicle technology issues (i.e., seat belts, air brakes, seat bags, and vehicle size).

Progress has been made in reducing deaths of children, teenagers, and adults in motor vehicle crashes in the 21st century. For example, the number of deaths of passenger vehicle drivers aged 16-19 years has dropped by 55% from 2004 (5,724 deaths) to 2013 (2,568 deaths) (14). Study of the Fatality Analysis Report System (FARS) by the CDC reveals that 9,644 passenger vehicle drivers aged 16 or 17 years were in fatal vehicle crashes from 2004 to 2008; there was a reduction of 38% of the annual population-based rate for these drivers involved in fatal crashes---from 27.1 per 100,000 in 2004 to 16.7 in 2008 (14). Progress in this endeavor has been noted in state after state where studied, such as in Alabama from 2000 to 2011, New Jersey from 2004 to 2008, New York State from 2004 to 2008 and others (272, 307).

Driving these remarkable reductions in death and injury are many factors such as stricter laws for teen drivers, delayed teen driver licensing, increased seat belt use, strict enforcement of laws on minimum legal drinking age, and augmented awareness by the public about risks of teen driving (272, 307). Children should always be properly restrained and safe transport between home and school should be assured (231).

Important measures seeking safety for young drivers and passengers include mandatory safety belt use, safer vehicles, antilock brakes, ignition lock devices, zero tolerance laws for alcohol, designated driver concepts, minimum drinking age laws, administrative per se laws, random drug and alcohol screening, avoidance of multiple passengers, and others (4-6, 253, 308). Implementation of basic safety measures for teen drivers led to a 40% decrease in fatal and police-reported crashes for 16 year old drivers between 1996 and 2005 (253). More states need to adopt strict laws which reduce underage drinking and decrease access that youth have for alcohol (309).

Implementation of the Graduated Licensing System (GLS) has saved young drivers' lives, though far too many continue to die (260). More research is needed as teenagers continue to die from MVCs and some fatalities involve teen drivers who had graduated from a GLS, wore seatbelts, and were not drug or alcohol-impaired (310). Modern technology is allowing study of kinematic risky driving based on data from accelerometers and global positioning systems (274). Legislative advocacy is need to strengthen and universalize GLS (311). Reduction in teenage fatal crashes can be made if we can establish robust, universal GLS laws in every state. Unfortunately, relatively minimal progress has been made in recent years in improving GLS legislation in many states (250, 307).

Progress can be made if various safety factors are enacted. For example, research notes lower teen driving death and injury rates in the State of Alabama from 2000 to 2011 and this lowering of morbidity and mortality in youth driving was related to various factors; these factors included stricter laws for teen drivers, delayed teen driver licensing, increased seat belt use, and augmented awareness by the public about risks of teen driving (215, 312). Progress will also come from studies on the novice driver based on solid scientific principles of research on various driving issues including distracted driving, multitasking while driving, mind wandering and other critical issues (Table 2) (4, 5, 42, 66, 231, 313-315).

Safety in all vehicles is need including cars, trucks, motorcycles, all-terrain vehicle (ATVs), bicycles, and others (4, 5, 18). Research is occurring on motor vehicle-bicycle interaction to improve the road safety for both operators of bicycles and motorcycles (316). There were 1,701 (ATV) rider deaths on public roads in the United States from 2007 to 2011 (17). Deaths on all-terrain vehicles (ATVs) can be reduced if drivers would not drive recklessly by speeding, driving while intoxicated, fail to wear helmets, and drive on roads even though ATVs are designed for off-road driving (17). Those on motorcycles and bicycles should always wear helmets (317, 318). It has been estimated that national mandatory helmet laws for motorcyclists would save $2.2 billion annually in prevention of mortality and hospital-involved morbidity (16).

Finally, it is ironic that deaths for drivers occurs in those who can afford to have cars in contrast to those from socioeconomic disadvantage who cannot afford to have such vehicles. Some members of society call for the development of low-cost, safe motor vehicles for all including those with limited fiscal resources (319). Since MVCs induce a high degree of death and injury for young teen drivers, the question for society is if all should be afforded such risks on the killing fields of American roads in the 21st century? However, a more critical concern is to reduce MVCs for all drivers from the many factors reviewed in this discussion including poor modeling from bad drivers and 21st century issue of distracted driving (320).

REFERENCES

[1] CDC and ICD-10. URL: http://wonder.cdc.gov/ucd-icd10.html.
[2] Centers for Disease Control and Prevention. Youth Risk Behavior Surveillance, United States, 1997. MMWR 1998;47(SS-3):1-89.
[3] Rosen DS, Xiangdong M, Blum RW: Adolescent health: Current trends and critical issues. State Art Rev Adolesc Med 1990;1(1):15-31.
[4] Patel DR. Greydanus DE, Rowlett JD. Romance with the automobile in the 20th century: implications for adolescents in a new millennium. Adolesc Med State Art Rev 2000;11(1):127-39.
[5] Greydanus DE, Merrick J. Post-traumatic stress disorder and motor vehicle accidents. J Pain Manage 2016;9(1):3-10.
[6] Margolis LH, Foss FD, Tolbert WG. Alcohol and motor vehicle-related deaths of children as passengers, pedestrians, and bicyclists. JAMA 2000;283(17):2245-8.
[7] United States Department of Transportation. National Highway Traffic Safety Administration. Traffic Safety Facts, 1998. URL: www.nhtsa.dot.gov.
[8] No authors. Years of potential life lost from unintentional injuries among persons aged 0-19 years—United States, 2000-2009. MMWR 2012;61(41):830-3.
[9] Durbin DR. Committee on Injury, Violence, and Poison Prevention. Pediatrics 2011;127(4):e1050-66.

[10] Quinlan K, Shults RA, Rudd RA. Child passenger deaths involving alcohol-impaired drivers. Pediatrics 2014;133(6):966-72.
[11] Fatalities in crashes involving young drivers, by person type and year, 2005-2014. Fatality Analysis Reporting System (FARSS) 2005-2013 Final File. 2014 Annual Report File. URL: https://crashstats.nhtsa.dot.govApi/Public/ViewPublication/812278.
[12] Motor vehicle traffic-related pedestrian deaths—United States, 2001-2010. MMWR 2013;62(15):277-82.
[13] Announcements: World Day of Remembrance for road traffic victims—November 18, 2012. MMWR 2012;61(45):928.
[14] No authors. Driving among high school students—United States, 2013. MMWR 2015;64(12):313-7.
[15] Mayr JM, Eder C, Berghold A, Wernig J, Khayati S, Ruppert-Kohlmayr A. Causes and consequences of pedestrian injuries in children. Eur J Pediatr 2003;162(3):184-90.
[16] Dua A, Wei S, Safarik J, Furlough C, Desai SS. National mandatory motorcycle helmet laws may save $2.2 billion annually: an inpatient and value of statistical life analysis. J Trauma Acute Care Surg 2015;78(6):1182-6.
[17] Williams AF, Oesch SL, McCartt AT, Teoh ER, Sims LB. On-road-all-terrain vehicle (ATV) fatalities in the United States. J Safety Res 2014; 50:117-23.
[18] Jung S, Xiao Q, Yoon Y. Evaluation of motorcycle safety strategies using the severity of injuries. Accid Anal Prev 2013;59:357-64.
[19] Bicyclist deaths associated with motor vehicle traffic—United States, 1975-2012. MMWR 2015;64(31):837-41.
[20] American Academy of Pediatrics. The teenage driver. Policy statement. Committee on Injury and Poison and Committee on Adolescence. Pediatrics 1996;98(5):987-90.
[21] Brown ID, Groeger JA: Risk perception and decision taking during the transition between novice and experienced driver status. Ergonomics 1988;31(4):585-597.
[22] Centers for Disease Control and Prevention: Youth Risk Behavior Surveillance, United States, 1997. MMWR 1998;47(SS-3):1-89.
[23] Centers for Disease Control and Prevention: Youth Risk Behavior Surveillance, United States, 1997. MMWR 1998;47(SS-3):1-89.
[24] Hofmann AD: Clinical assessment and management of health risk behaviors in adolescents. State Art Rev Adol Med 1990;1(1):33-44.
[25] Hofmann AD. Adolescent growth and development. In: Hofmann SD, Greydanus DE, eds. Adolescent medicine, third edition. Stamford, CT: Appleton Lange, 1997:10-22.
[26] Insurance Institute for Highway Safety, Arlington, VA, and Traffic Injury Research Foundation of Canada, Ontario, Canada: Graduated Licensing: A Blueprint for North America. 1999.
[27] Williams AF: Graduated licensing comes to the United States. Inj Prev 1999;5:133-5.
[28] United States Department of Transportation T. Risk perception and age-specific accidents of young drivers. National Highway Traffic Safety Administration, Saving

Teenage Lives, 1999. URL: http://www.nhtsa.dot.gov/people/injury/newdriver/Save Teens/sect1.html.
[29] United States Department of Transportation. National Highway Traffic Safety Administration. Traffic Safety Facts, 1998. URL: www.nhtsa.dot.gov.
[30] Evans L: Traffic safety and the driver. New York: Van Nostrand Reinhold, 1991.
[31] COMSIS Corp Report: Understanding youthful risk taking and driving, Interim report, Contract No: DRNH22-93-C-05182. Prepared by COMSIS Corporation, Silver Spring, MD, and The Johns Hopkins University, Baltimore, MD. Washington, DC: US Department Transportation, 1995.
[32] Steinbeck K, Towns S, Bennett D. Adolescent and young adult medicine is a special and specific area of medical practice. J Paediatr Child Health 2014;50(6):427-31.
[33] Dekker DK, Kotwal BM, Lerner ND. Understanding driver performance variability and perception of risk. Technical Report for Federal Highway Administration. 1994.
[34] DeJoy DM. An examination of gender differences in traffic accident risk perception. Accid Anal Prev 1992;24(3):237-46.
[35] Lambert N. Analysis of driving histories of ADHD subjects. Cooperative Agreement No. DTNH22-94-H-05320). Unpublished report. Washington, DC: Department Transportation, National Highway Traffic Safety Administration, 1995.
[36] Irwin CE Jr. The theoretical concept of at-risk adolescents. State Art Rev Adol Med 1990;1(1):1-14.
[37] Hatfield J, Fernandes R, Job FF. Thrill and adventure seeking as a modifier of the relationship of perceived risk with risky driving among young drivers. Accid Anal Prev 2014;62:223-9.
[38] Hanna CL, Hasselberg M, Laflamme L. Young, unlicensed drivers and fatal road traffic crashes in the USA in the past decade. A neglected public health issue. Inj Prev 2014;20(1):54-6.
[39] Begg DJ, Langley JD, Brookland RL, Ameratunga S, Gulliver P. Pre-licensed driving experiences and car crash involvement during the learner and restricted, license stages of graduated driver licensing: Findings from the New Zealand drivers study. Accid Anal Prev 2014;62:153-60.
[40] Keating DP, Halpern-Felsher BL. Adolescent drivers: a developmental perspective on risk, proficiency, and safety. Am J Prev Med 2008;35(3 Suppl):S272-7.
[41] Ivers R, Senserrick T, Boufous S, Stevenson M, Chen HY, Woodward M, et al. Novice drivers' risky driving behavior, risk perception, and crash risk: findings from the DRIVE study. Am J Publ Health 2009;99(9):1638-44.
[42] Scott-Parker B, Watson B, King MJ, Hyde MK. Young and unlicensed: risky driving before entering the licensing system. Traffic Inj Prev 2012;13(3):213-8.
[43] Shope JT, Bingham CR. Teen driving: motor-vehicle crashes and factors that contribute. Am J Prev Med 2008;35(Suppl 3):S261-71.
[44] Gonzales MM, Dickinson LM, DiGuiseppi C, Lowenstein SR. Student drivers: a study of fatal motor vehicle crashes involving 16-year-old drivers. Ann Emerg Med 2005;45(2):140-6.
[45] Roman GD, Poulter D, Barker E, McKenna FP, Rowe R. Novice drivers' individual trajectories of driver behavior over the first three years of driving. Accid Anal Prev 2015;82:61-9.

[46] Guinosso SA, Johnson SB, Schultheis MT, Graefe AC, Bishai DM. Neurocognitive correlates of young drivers' performance in a driving simulator. J Adolesc Health 2016;58(4):467-73.
[47] Pope CN, Ross LA, Stavrinos D. Association between executive function and problematic adolescent driving. J Dev Behav Pediatr 2016;37(9):702-711.
[48] DeJoy DM. The optimism bias and traffic accident risk perception. Accid Anal Prev 1989;21(4):333-40.
[49] Farrow JA. Personality factors associated with driving while intoxicated: A comparison study of adolescent drivers. J Alcohol Drug 1988;34(2):21-32.
[50] Foss RD, Evanson KR. Effectiveness of graduated driver licensing in reducing motor vehicle crashes. Am J Prev Med 1999;16 (1S):47-56.
[51] Lerner N, Williams A, Sedney C. Risk perception in highway driving. Contract No. DTFH61-85-C-00143. Washington, DC. Department Transportation, Federal Highway Administration, 1988.
[52] Mayhew DR, Simpson HM. Young drivers and novice drivers. New to the Road: similar problems and solutions? Ottawa, ON: Traffic Injury Research Foundation Canada, 1990.
[53] Sivak M, Soler J, Tränkle U, Spagnhol JM. Cross-cultural differences in driver risk-perception. Accid Anal Prev 1989;21(4):355-62.
[54] Selzer SC. Normal psychological development: Theories and concepts. In: Greydanus DE, Wolraich ML, eds. Behavioral pediatrics. New York: Springer, 1992:1-15.
[55] Cairney PT. An exploratory study of risk estimates of driving situations. Proceedings of the ARRP Conference 1982;11(5):233-240.
[56] Finn P, Bragg WE: Perception of the risk of an accident by young and older drivers. Accid Anal Prev 1986;18(4):289-98.
[57] Kazden AE. Conduct disorder in childhood and adolescence. Newbury Park, CA: Sage, 1987.
[58] Jonah B. Accident risk and risk-taking behavior among young drivers. Accid Anal Prev 1986;18(4):255-71.
[59] Farrow JA. Young driver risk taking: A description of dangerous driving situations among 16- to 19-year old drivers. Int J Addict 1987;22:1255-67.
[60] Barkely RA, Guevremont DC, Anastopoulos AD, DuPaul GJ, Shelton TL. Driving-related risks and outcomes of attention deficit hyperactivity disorder in adolescents and young adults: A 3-to 5- year follow-up survey. Pediatrics 1993;92(2):212-8.
[61] Stafford Sewall AA, Whetsel Borzendowski SA, Tyrrell RA. The accuracy of drivers' judgments of the effects of headlight glare on their own visual acuity. Perception 2014;43(11):1203-13.
[62] Taubman-Ben Ari O, Katz-Ben-Ami L. The contribution of family climate for road safety and social environment to the reported driving behavior of young drivers. Accid Anal Prev 2012;47:1-10.
[63] Mirman JH, Curry AE, Winston FK, Fisher Thiel MC, Pfeiffer MR, Rogers R, et al. Parental influence on driver licensure in adolescents: a randomized control trial. Health Psychol 2016 Dec 12. [Epub ahead of print].

[64] Phebo L, Dellinger AM: Young driver involvement in fatal motor vehicle crashes and trends in risk behaviors, United States, 1988-95. Inj Prev 1998;4:284-7.
[65] Houwing S, Twisk D. Nothing good ever happened after midnight: observed exposure and alcohol use during weekend nights among young male drivers carrying passengers in a late licensing country. Accid Anal Prev 2015;75:61-8.
[66] Scott-Parker B, Oviedo-Trespalacios O. Young driver risky behavior and predictors of crash risk in Australia, New Zealand and Columbia: Same but different? Accid Anal Prev 2016;99(Pt A):30-8.
[67] Greydanus DE, Kaplan G, Baxter LE Sr, Patel DR, Feucht CL. Cannabis: The never-ending, nefarious nepenthe of the 21st century: What should the clinician know? Dis Mon 2015;61(4):118-75.
[68] Warren RA, Simpson HM. The young driver paradox. Ottawa, ON: Traffic Injury Foundation Canada, 1976.
[69] Summala H. Young driver accidents: Risk taking or failure of skills? Alcohol Drugs Driving 1987;3(304):79-91.
[70] Machin MA, Sankey KS. Relationship between young drivers' personality characteristics, risk perceptions, and driving behavior. Accid Anal Prev 2008;40(2):541-7.
[71] Durbin DR, Mirman JH, Curry AE, Wang W, Fisher Thiel MC, et al. Driver errors of learner teens: frequency, nature, and their association with practice. Accid Anal Prev 2014;72:433-9.
[72] McDonald CC, Goodwin AH, Pradhan AK, Romoser MR, Williams AF. A review of hazard anticipation training programs for young drivers. J Adolesc Heatlh 2015;57(Suppl 1):S15-23.
[73] Hoffman Y, Rosenbloom T. Driving experience moderates the effect of implicit versus explicit threat priming on hazard perception test. Accid Anal Prev 2016;92:82-8.
[74] Curry AE, Hafetz J, Kallan MJ, Winston FK, Durbin DR. Prevalence of teen driver errors leading to serious motor vehicle crashes. Accid Anal Prev 2011;43(4):1285-90.
[75] Parker D, Manstead ASR, Stradling SG, Reason JT. Determinants of intention to commit driving violations. Accid Anal Prev 1992;24(2):117-31.
[76] Mirman JH, Curry AE. Racing with friends: resistance to peer influence, gist, and specific risk beliefs. Accid Anal Prev 2016;96;180-4.
[77] Evans L, Wasielewski P. Risky driving related to driver and vehicle characteristics. Accid Anal Prev 1983;5(2):121-136.
[78] Farrow JA. Young driver risk taking: A description of dangerous driving situations among 16- to 19-year old drivers. Int J Addict 1987;22:1255-67.
[79] Aeron-Thomas AS, Hess S. Red-light cameras for prevention of road traffic crashes. Cochrane Database Syst Rev 2005;2:CD003862.
[80] Simons-Morton BG, Ouimet MC, Chen R, Klauer SG, Lee SE, Wang J, et al. Peer influence predicts speeding prevalence among teenage drivers. J Safety Res 2012;43(5-6):397-403.

[81] Scott-Parker B, Hyde MK, Watson B, King MJ. Speeding by novice drivers: What can personal characteristics and psychosocial theory add to our understanding? Accid Anal Prev 2013;50:242-50.
[82] Braitman KA, Kirley BB, McCartt AT, Chaudhary NK. Crashes of novice teenage drivers: characteristics and contributing factors. J Safety Res 2008;39(1):47-54.
[83] Finn P, Bragg WE. Perception of the risk of an accident by young and older drivers. Accid Anal Prev 1986;18(4):289-98.
[84] Ellison AB, Greaves SP. Speeding in urban environments: Are the time savings worth the risk? Accid Anal Prev 2015;85:239-47.
[85] Rowe R, Andrews E, Harris PR, Armitage CJ, McKenna FP, Norman P. Identifying beliefs underlying pre-drivers' intentions to take risks: An application of the Theory of Planned Behavior. Accid Anal Prev 2016;89:49-56.
[86] Mirman JH, Curry AE. Racing with friends: resistance to peer influence, gist, and specific risk beliefs. Accid Anal Prev 2016;96;180-4.
[87] Hosking SG, Young KL, Regan MA. The effects of messaging on young drivers. Hum Factors 2009;51(4):582-92.
[88] O'Brien NP, Goodwin AH, Foss RD. Talking and texting among teenage drivers: a glass half empty or half full? Traffic Inj Prev 2010;11(6):549-54.
[89] Kann L, McManus T, Harris WA, Shanklin SL, Flint KH, Hawkins J et al. Youth Risk Behavior Surveillance, 2015. MMWR 2016;65(6):1-174.
[90] Bakiri S, Galéra C, Lagarde E, Laborey M, Contrand B, Ribéreau-Gayon R, et al. Distraction and driving: results from a case-control responsibility study of traffic crash injured drivers interviewed at the emergency room. Accid Anal Prev 2013;59:588-92.
[91] Adeola R, Omorogbe A, Johnson A. Get the message: A teen distracted program. J Trauma Nurs 2016;23(6);312-20.
[92] Tractinsky N, Ram ES, Shinar D. To call or not to call—that is the question (while driving). Accid Anal Prev 2013;56:59-70.
[93] Pope CN, Bell TR, Stavrinos D. Mechanisms behind distracted driving behavior: The role of age and executive function in the engagement of distracted driving. Accid Anal Prev 2017;98:123-9.
[94] Simmons SM, Hicks A, Caird JK. Safety-critical event risk associated with cell phone tasks as measured in naturalistic driving studies; A systematic review and meta-analysis. Accid Anal Prev 2016;87:161-9.
[95] Dozza M, Flannagan CA, Saver JR. Real-world effects of using a phone while driving on lateral and longitudinal control of vehicles. J Safety Res 2015;55: 81-7.
[96] Farmer CM, Klauer SG, McClafferty JA, Guo F. Relationship of near-crash/crash risk to time spent on a cell phone while driving. Traffic Inj Prev 2015;16(8):792-800.
[97] Sullman MJ, Prat F, Tasci DK. A roadside study of observable driver distractions. Traffic Inj Prev 2015;16(6):552-7.
[98] Braitman KA, McCartt AT. National reported patterns of driver cell phone use in the United States. Traffic Inj Prev 2010;11(6):543-8.
[99] Foss RD, Goodwin AH, McCartt AT, Hellinga LA. Short-term effects of a teenage driver cell phone restriction. Accid Anal Prev 2009;41(3):419-24.

[100] Ehsani JP, Bingham CR, Ionides E, Childers D. The impact of Michigan's text messaging restriction on motor vehicle crashes. J Adolesc Health 54(Suppl 5):S68-74.
[101] McCartt AT, Kidd DG, Teoh ER. Driver cellphone and texting bans in the United States: evidence of effectiveness. Ann Adv Automot Med 2014;58:99-114.
[102] Havashi Y, Russo CT, Wirth O. Texting while driving as impulsive choice: a behavioral economic analysis. Accid Anal Prev 2015;83:182-9.
[103] Tefft BC, Williams AF, Grabowski JG. Teen driver risk in relation to age and number of passengers, United States, 2007-2010. Traffic Inj Prev 2013;14(3):283-92.
[104] Ouimet MC, Pradhan AK, Simons-Morton BG, Divekar G, Mehranian H, Fisher DL. The effect of male teenage passengers on male teenage drivers; findings from a driving simulator study. Accid Anal Prev 2013;58:132-9.
[105] Foss RD, Goodwin AH. Distracted driver behaviors and distracting conditions among adolescent drivers: findings from a naturalistic driving study. J Adolesc Health 2014;54(Suppl 5):S50-60.
[106] Pradhan AK, Li K, Bingham CR, Simons-Morton BG, Ouimet MC, Shope JT. Peer passenger influences on male adolescent drivers' visual scanning behavior during simulated driving. J Adolesc Health 2014;54(5 Suppl):S42-9.
[107] Heck KE, Carlos RM. Passenger distractions among adolescent drivers. J Safety Res 2008;39(4):437-43.
[108] Delgado MK, Wanner KJ, McDonald C. Adolescent cellphone use while driving: an overview of the literature and promising future directions for prevention. Media Commun 2016;4(3):79-89.
[109] Parr MN, Ross LA, McManus B, Bishop HJ, Wittig SM, Stavrinos D. Differential impact of personality traits on distracted driving behaviors in teens and older adults. Accid Anal Prev 2016;92:107-12.
[110] Li Q, Tav R. Improving drivers' knowledge of road rules using digital games. Accid Anal Prev 2014;65.8-10.
[111] Simons-Morton BG, Guo F, Klauer SG, Ehsani JP, Pradhan AK. Keep your eyes on the road: young driver crash risk increases according to duration of distraction. J Adolesc Health 2014;54(Suppl 5):S61-7.
[112] McDonald CC, Sommers MS. Teen drivers' perceptions of inattention and cell phone use while driving. Traffic Inj Prev 2015;16(Suppl 2):S52-8.
[113] Gauld CS, Lewis IM, White KM, Watson B. Key beliefs influencing young drivers' engagement with social interactive technology on their smartphones: a qualitative study. Traffic Inj Prev 2016;17(2):128-33.
[114] Carter PM, Bingham CR, Zakraisek JS, Shope JT, Sayer TB. Social norms and risk perception: predictors of distracted driving behavior among novice adolescent drivers. J Adolesc Health 2014;54(Suppl 5):S32-41.
[115] Raymond Bingham C, Zakraisek JS, Almani F, Shope JT, Saver TB. Do as I say, not as I do: Distracted driving behavior of teens and their parents. J Safety Res 2015;55:21-9.

[116] Soccolich SA, Fitch GM, Perez MA, Hanowski RJ. Comparing handheld and hands-free cell phone usage behaviors while driving. Traffic Inj Prev 2014;15 Suppl 1:S21-6.
[117] Mirman JH, Albert D, Jacobsohn LS, Winston FK. Factors associated with adolescents' propensity to drive with multiple passengers and to engage in risky driving behaviors. J Adolesc Health 2012;50(6):634-40.
[118] Lierena LE, Aronow KV, Macleod J, Bard M, Salzman S, Greene W, et al. An evidence-based review: distracted driver. J Trauma Acute Care Surg 2015;78(1):147-52.
[119] Huisingh C, Griffin R, McGwin G Jr. The prevalence of distraction among passenger vehicle drivers: a roadside observational approach. Traffic Inj Prev 2015;16(2):140-8.
[120] Ferdinand AO, Menachemi N, Sen B, Blackburn JL, Morrisey M, Nelson L. Impact of texting laws on motor vehicular fatalities in the United States. Am J Public Health 2014;104(8):1370-7.
[121] Rudisill TM, Zhu M. The association between states' texting regulations and the prevalence of texting while driving among U.S. high school students. Ann Epidemiol 2015;25(12);888-93.
[122] Zhu M, Rudisill TM, Heeringa S, Swedler D, Redelmeier DA. The association between handheld phone bans and the prevalence of handheld phone conversations among young drivers in the United States. Ann Epidemiol 2016;26(12):833-7.
[123] Creaser JI, Edwards CJ, Morris NL, Donath M. Are cellular phone blocking applications effective for novice teen drivers? J Safety Res 2015;54:75-8.
[124] Buckley L, Chapman RL, Sheehan M. Young driver distraction: state of the evidence and directions for behavior change programs. J Adolesc Health 2014;54(Suppl 5):S12-21.
[125] Overton TL, Rives RE, Hecht C, Shafi S, Gandhi RR. Distracted driving: prevalence, problems, and prevention. Int J Inj Contr Saf Promot 2015;22(3):187-92.
[126] Xiong H, Bao S, Saver J, Kato K. Examination of drivers' cell phone use behavior at intersections by using naturalistic driving data. J Safety Res 2015;54:59-93.
[127] Tivesten E, Dozza M. Driving context influences drivers' decision to engage in visual-manual phone tasks: evidence from a naturalistic driving study. J Safety Res 2015;53:87-96.
[128] Sanbonmatsu DM, Stayer DL, Behrends AA, Ward N, Watson JM. Why drivers use cell phones and support legislation to restrict this practice. Accid Anal Prev 2016;92:22-33.
[129] Ouimet MC, Pradhan AK, Brooks-Russell A, Ehsani JP, Berbiche D, Simons-Morton BG. Young drivers and their passengers: a systematic review of epidemiologic studies on crash risk. J Adolesc Health 2015;57(Suppl 1):S24-35.
[130] McDonald CC, Sommers MS. "Good passengers and not good passengers:" Adolescent drivers' perceptions about inattention and peer passengers. J Pediatr Nurs 2016;31(6):e375-e382.
[131] Centers for Disease Control and Prevention. Vital signs: drinking and driving among high school students aged =16 years-United States, 1991-2011. MMWR 2012;61:796-800.

[132] Azofeifa A, Mattison ME, Lyerla R. Driving under the influence of alcohol, marijuana, and alcohol and marijuana combined among persons aged 16-25 years- United States, 2002-2014. MMWR 2015;64(48):1325-9.
[133] Mayhew DR, Donelson AC, Beirness DJ, Simpson HM. Youth alcohol, and relative risk of crash involvement. Accid Anal Prev 1986;18(4):273-87.
[134] Zador PL. Alcohol-related relative risk of fatal driver injuries in relation to driver age and sex. J Study Alcohol 1991;52:302-10.
[135] Hultgren BA, Scaglione NM, Cleveland MJ, Turrisi R. Examination of a dual-process model predicting riding with drinking drivers. Alcohol Clin Exp Res 2015;39(6):1075-82.
[136] Ewing BA, Tucker JS, Miles JN, Shih RA, Kulesza M, Pedersen ER, et al. Early substance use and subsequent DWI in adolescents. Pediatrics 2015;136(5):868-75.
[137] Harris SK, Johnson JK, Sherritt L, Copelas S, Rappo MA, Wilson CR. Putting adolescents at risk: Riding with drinking drivers who are adults in the home. J Stud Alcohol Drugs 2017;78(1):146-51.
[138] Williams AF, Tefft BC. Characteristics of teen-with-teens fatal crashes in the United States, 2005-2010. J Safety Res 2014;48:37-42.
[139] O'Malley PM, Johnston LD: Drinking and driving among US high school seniors, 1984-1997. Am J Publ Health 1999;89(5):678-84.
[140] United States Department of Transportation. National Highway Safety Administration. Graduated driver licensing system for young drivers: Guidelines for motor vehicle administrators. Washington, DC. NHTSA. DOT HS-808-331, 1996.
[141] Klepp KI, Perry CL: Adolescents, drinking, and driving: Who does it and why? In: Wilson J, Mann RE, eds. Drinking and driving: advances in research and prevention. New York: Guilford, 1990:42-67.
[142] Elander J, West R, French D. Behavioral correlates of individual differences in road-traffic crash risk: An examination of methods and findings. Psychol Bull 1993;113(2):279-94.
[143] Vegega M, Klitzner M. What have we learned about youth anti-drinking-driving programs? Eval Prog Plan 1988;11:203-17.
[144] Williams AF, Preusser DF, Ferguson SA, et al: Analysis of the fatal crash involvements of 15-year-old drivers. J Safety Res1997;28:49-54.
[145] Teale D, Marks V. A fatal motor-car accident and cannabis use. Investigation by radioimmunoassay. Lancet 1976;1:884-5.
[146] Greydanus DE, Apple R. Cannabis and driving. In: Cabana M, ed. Year book of pediatrics. Philadelphia, PA: Elsevier Mosby, 2015:2-4.
[147] Li MC, Brady JE, DiMaggio CJ, Lusardi AR, Tzong KY, Li G. Marijuana use and motor vehicle crashes. Epidemiol Rev 2012;34:65-72.
[148] Sewell RA, Poling J, Sofuoglu M. The effect of cannabis compared with alcohol on driving. Am J Addict 2009;18(3):185-93.
[149] Cartwright J, Asbridge M. Passengers' decisions to ride with a driver under the influence of either alcohol or cannabis. J Stud Alcohol Drugs 2011;72(1):86-95.
[150] Asbridge M, Hayden JA, Cartwright JL. Acute cannabis consumption and motor vehicle collision risk: systemic review of observational studies and meta-analysis. BMJ 2012 Feb 9;344:e536.doi:10:1136/bmj.e536.

[151] Johnson MB, Kelley-Baker G, Voas RB, Lacey JH. The prevalence of cannabis-involved driving in California. Drug Alcohol Depend 2012;123(1-3):105-9.
[152] Kuypers KP, Legrand SA, Ramaekers JG, Verstraete AG. A case-control study estimating accident for alcohol, medicines, and illegal drugs. PLoS One 2012;7(8):e43496. doi: 10.1371/journal.pone.0043496.
[153] Downey LA, King R, Papafotiou K, Swann P, Ogden E, Boorman M, et al. The effects of cannabis and alcohol on simulated driving: influences of dose and experience. Accid Anal Prev 2013;50:879-86.
[154] Bergamaschi MM, Karschner El, Goodwin RS, Scheidweiler KB, Hirvonen J, Queiroz RH, et al. Impact of prolonged cannabinoid excretion in chronic daily cannabis smokers' blood on per se drugged driving laws. Clin Chem 2013;59(3):519-26.
[155] Neavyn MJ, Blohm E, Babu KM, Bird SB. Medical marijuana and driving: a review. J Med Toxicol 2014;10(3):269-70.
[156] Poulsen H, Moar R, Pirie R. The culpability of drivers killed in New Zealand road crashes and their use of alcohol and other drugs. Accid Anal Prev 2014;67:119-28.
[157] Lenné MG, Dietze PM, Triggs TJ, Walmsley S, Murphy B, Redman JR. The effects of cannabis and alcohol on simulated arterial driving: influences of driving experiences and task demand. Accid Anal Prev 2010;42:859-66.
[158] Hartman RL, Huestis MA. Cannabis effects on driving skills. Clin Chem 2013;59:478-92.
[159] Hartman RL, Brown TL, Milavetz G, Spurgin A, Pierce RS, Gorelick DA, et al. Cannabis effects on driving lateral control with and without alcohol. Drug Alcohol Depend 2015;154:25-37.
[160] Whitehill JM, Rivera FP, Moreno MA. Marijuana-using drivers, alcohol-using drivers, and their passengers: prevalence and risk factors among underage college students. JAMA Pediatr 2014;168(7):618-24.
[161] Volkow ND, Baler RD, Compton WH, Weiss SR. Adverse health effects of marijuana use. N Engl J Med 2014;370:2219-27.
[162] National Institute on Drug Abuse. Research report series: marijuana. Publication No. 15-3859. Bethesda, MD: National Institutes of Health, National Institute on Drug Use, 2015. URL: https://www.drugabuse.gov/sites/default/files/mjrrs 4 15.pdf.
[163] Berning A, Compton R, Wochinger K. Results of the 2013-2014 National Roadside Survey of Alcohol and Drug Use by Drivers, Report No. DOT HS 812 118. Washington, DC: Department Transportation, National Highway Traffic Safety Administration, 2015.
[164] Smart R, Stoduto G, Mann R, Adlaf E. Road rage experience and behavior: vehicle, exposure, and driver factors. Traffic Inj Prev 2004;5(4):343-8.
[165] Mann RE, Zhao J, Stoduto G, Adlaf EM, Smart RG, Donovan JE. Road rage and collision involvement. Am J Health Behav 2007;31(4):384-91.
[166] Stephens AN, Sullman MJ. Trait predictors of aggression and crash-related behaviors across drivers from the United Kingdom and the Irish Republic. Risk Anal 2015;35(9):1730-45.
[167] Sagar R, Mehta M, Chugh G. Road rage: an exploratory study on aggressive driving experience on Indian roads. Int J Soc Psychiatry 2013;59(4):407-12.

[168] Esiyok B, Yasak Y, Korkusuz I. Anger expression on the road: validity and reliability of the driving anger expression inventory. Turk Psikiyatri Derg 2007;18(3);231-43. [Turkish].
[169] Kovácscová N, Rošková E. Lajunen T. Forgiveness, anger, and hostility in aggressive driving. Accid Anal Prev 2014;62:303-8.
[170] Ilie G, Mann RE, Ialomiteanu A, Adlaf EM, Hamilton H, Wickens CM, et al. Traumatic brain injury, driver aggression and motor vehicle collisions in Canadian adults. Accid Anal Prev 2015;81:1-7.
[171] Fierro I, Morales C, Alvarez FJ. Alcohol use, illicit drug use, and road rage. J Stud Alcohol Drugs 2011;72(2):185-93.
[172] Fong G, Frost D, Stansfeld S. Road rage: A psychiatric phenomenon? Soc Psychiatry Psychiatr Epidemiol 2001;36(6):277-86.
[173] Benavidez DC, Flores AM, Fierro I, Alvarez FJ. Road rage among drug dependent patients. Accid Anal Prev 2013;50:848-53.
[174] Sansone RA, Lam C, Widerman MW: Road rage: relationships with borderline personality and driving citations. Int J Psychiatry Med 2010; 40(1):21-9.
[175] Sansone RA, Leung JS, Wiederman MW. Driving citations and aggressive behavior. Traffic Inj Prev 2012;13(3):337-40.
[176] Richards TL, Deffenbacher JL, Rosén LA, Barkley RA, Rodricks T. Driving anger and driving behavior in adults with ADHD. J Atten Disord 2006;10(1):54-64.
[177] Lucidi F, Giannini AM, Sgalla R, Mallia L, Devoto A, Reichmann S. Young novice driver subtypes: relationship to driving violations, errors and lapses. Accid Anal Prev 2010;42(6):1689-96.
[178] Parkinson B. Anger on and off the road. Br J Psychol 2001;92(Pt 3):507-26.
[179] Sivak M. Homicide rate as a predictor of traffic fatality rate. Traffic Inj Prev 2009;10(6):511-2.
[180] Roberts LD, Indermaur DW. The "homogamy" of road rage revisited. Violence Vict 2008;23(6):758-72.
[181] Dula CS, Geller ES. Risky, aggressive, or emotional driving: addressing the need for consistent communication in research. J Safety Res 2003;34(5):559-66.
[182] Johnson MB, McKnight S. Warning drivers about potential congestion as a means to reduce frustration-driven aggressive driving. Traffic Inj Prev 2009;10(4):354-60.
[183] Stephens AN, Groeger JA. Anger-congruent behavior transfers across driving situations. Cogn Emot 2011;25(8):1423-38.
[184] Taubman-Ben-Ari O, Kaplan S, Lotan T, Prato CG. Parents' and peers' contribution to risky driving of male teen drivers. Accid Anal Prev 2015;78:81-6.
[185] Asbridge M, Smart RG, Mann RE. Can we prevent road rage? Trauma Violence Abuse 2006;7(2):109-21.
[186] Deffenbacher JL, Lynch RS, Filetti LB, Dahlen ER, Oetting ER. Anger, aggression, risky behavior, and crash-related outcomes in three groups of drivers. Behav Res Ther 2003;41(3):333-49.
[187] Deffenbacher JL, Richards TL, Filetti LB, Lynch RS. Angry drivers: a test of state-trait theory. Violence Vict 2005;20(4):455-69.
[188] Fruhen LS, Flin R. Car driver attitudes, perceptions of social normal and aggressive driving behavior toward cyclists. Accid Anal Prev 2015;83:162-70.

[189] Drazkowski J. An overview of epilepsy and driving. Epilepsia 2007;48 Suppl 9:10-2.
[190] Tatum WO, Worley AV, Selenica ML. Disobedience and driving in patients with epilepsy. Epilepsy Behav 2012;23(1):30-5.
[191] Cox DJ, Gonder-Frederick LA, Shepard JA, Campbell LK, Vajda KA. Driving safety: concerns and experiences of parents of adolescent drivers with type 1 diabetes. Pediatr Diabetes 2012;13(6):506-9.
[192] Tefft BC. Prevalence of motor vehicle crashes involving drowsy drivers, United States, 1999-2008. Accid Anal Prev 2012;45:180-6.
[193] Martiniuk AL, Senserrick T, Lo S, Williamson A, Du W, Grunstein RR, et al. Sleep-deprived young drivers and the risk for crash: the DRIVE prospective cohort study. JAMA Pediatr 2013;167(7):647-55.
[194] Wheaton AG, Chapman DP, Presley-Cantrell LR, Croft JB. Drowsy driving --19 states and the District of Columbia, 2009-2010. MMWR 2013;61(51):1033-7.
[195] Wheaton AG, Shults RA, Chapman DP, Ford ES, Croft JB. Drowsy driving and risk behaviors—10 states and Puerto Rico, 2011-2012. MMWR 2014;63(26):557-62.
[196] Greydanus DE, Feucht C. Sleep disorders and sleep patterns in adolescents. J Altern Med Res 2012;4(2):129-47.
[197] Greydanus DE. Intellectual disability: sleep disorders. J Altern Med Res 2015;7(4):33-40.
[198] Danner F, Phillips B. Adolescent sleep, school start times, and teen motor vehicle crashes. J Clin Sleep Med 2008;4(6):533-5.
[199] Verona RD, Szklo-Coxe M, Lamichhane R, Ware JC, McNallen A, Leszczyszyn D. Adolescent crash rates and school start times in two central Virginia counties, 2009-2011: a follow-up study to a southeastern Virginia study, 2007-2008. J Clin Sleep Med 2014;10(11):1169-77.
[200] George CF. Sleep apnea, alertness, and motor vehicle crashes. Am J Respir Crit Care Med 2007;176(10):954-6.
[201] Karimi M, Hedner J, Lombardi C, Mcnicholas WT, Penzel T, Riha RL, et al. Driving habits and risk factors for traffic accidents among sleep apnea patients—a European multi-centre cohort study. J Sleep Res 2014;23(6):689-99.
[202] ay JF, Porter BE, Ware JC. The deterioration of driving performance over time in drivers with untreated sleep apnea. Accid Anal Prev 2016;89;95-102.
[203] Greydanus DE, Pratt HD, Patel DR: Attention deficit hyperactivity disorder across the lifespan. Disease-a-Month 2007;53(2):65-132.
[204] Huang P, Kao T, Curry AE, Durbin DR. Factors associated with driving in teens with autism spectrum disorders. J Dev Behav Pediatr 2012;33(1):70-4.
[205] Classen S, Monahan M, Brown KE, Hernandez S. Driving indicators in teens with attention deficit hyperactivity disorder and/or autism spectrum disorder. Can J Occup Ther 2013;80(5):274-83.
[206] Cox SM, Cox DJ, Kofler MJ, Moncrief MA, Johnson RJ, Lambert AE, et al. Driving simulator performance in novice drivers with autism spectrum disorder: The role of executive functions and basic motor skills. J Autism Dev Disord 2016;46(4)1379-91.
[207] Barkley RA. Commentary: One way attention-deficit/hyperactivity disorder can be life threatening: a travelogue on Nicholas et al. ((2016). J Child Psychol Psychiatr 2016;57(2):149-51.

[208] Barkley RA. Driving impairments in teens and adults with attention-deficit/hyperactivity disorder. Psychiatr Clin North Am 2004; 27(2):233-60.
[209] Aduen PA, Kofler MJ, Cox DJ, Sarver DE, Lunsford E. Motor vehicle driving in high incidence psychiatric disability: comparison of drivers with ADHD, depression, and no known psychopathology. J Psychiatr Res 2015;64:59-66.
[210] Fabiano GA, Schatz NK, Hulme KF, Morris KL, Vujnovic RK, Willoughby MT, et al. Positive bias in teenage drivers with ADHD within a simulated driving task. J Atten Disord 2015 Dec 4. pii: 1087054715616186.
[211] Merkel RL Jr., Nichols JQ, Fellers JC, Hidalgo P, Martinez LA, Putziger I, et al. Comparison of on-road driving between young adults with and without ADHD. J Atten Disord 2016;20(3):260-9.
[212] Fabiano GA, Schatz NK, Morris KL, Willoughby MT, Vujnovic RK, Hulme KF, et al. Efficacy of a family-focused intervention for young drivers with attention-deficit hyperactivity disorder. J Consult Clin Psychol 2016;84(12):1078-93.
[213] Lorini C, Pieralli F, Mersi A, Cecconi R, Garofalo G, Santini MG, et al. Comparison of self-reported and observed prevalence of seat belt and helmet use in Florence. Ann Ig 2014;26(6):499-506.
[214] Rivara FP: Effectiveness of primary and secondary enforced seat belt laws. Am J Prev Med 1999;16:30-9.
[215] Monroe K, Irons E, Crew M, Norris J, Nichols M, King WD. Trends in Alabama in teen driving death and injury. J Trauma Acute Care Surg 2014;77(3 Suppl 1):S51-4.
[216] Han GM, Newmyer A, Qu M. Seat belt use to save face: impact on drivers' body region and nature of injury in motor vehicle crashes. Traffic Inj Prev 2015;16(6):605-10.
[217] Chen GX, Collins JW, Sieber WK, Pratt SG, Rodríguez-Acosta RL, Lincoln JE, et al. Vital signs: seat belt use among long-haul truck drivers—United States, 2010. MMWR 2015;64(08):217-21.
[218] Goldzweig IA, Levine RS, Schlundt D, Bradley R, Jones GD, Zoorob RJ, et al. Improving seat belt use among teen drivers: findings from a service-learning approach. Accid Anal Prev 2013;59:71-5.
[219] Bao S, Xiong H, Buonarosa ML, Saver JR. Using naturalistic driving data to examine drivers' seatbelt use behavior: Comparison between teens and adults. J Safety Res 2015;54:69-73.
[220] Elliott MR, Ginsburg KR, Winston FK. Unlicensed teenage drivers: who are they, and how do they behave when they are behind the wheel? Pediatrics 2008;122(5):e994-1000.
[221] Donahue WA: Issues of risk in adult and teen safety belt use. Alcohol Drugs Driving 1988;4(3-4):297-304.
[222] Murphy JM. Child passenger safety. J Pediatr Health Care 1998; 12(3):130-8.
[223] Evans L, Gerrish PH: Antilock brakes and risk of front and rear impact in two-vehicle crashes. Accid Anal Prev 1996;28:315-23.
[224] Rivara FP: Systematic reviews of strategies to prevent motor vehicle injuries. Am J Prev Med 1999;16:1-5.
[225] Rivara FP, Rivara MB, Bartol K: Dad, May I have the Keys? Factors influencing which vehicles teenagers drive. Pediatrics 1998;102(5):e57.

[226] Shen S, Nevens DM. The effects of age, gender, and crash types on drivers' injury-related health care costs. Accid Anal Prev 2015;77:82-90.
[227] Evans L, Frick MC: Car size or mass: Which has greater influence on fatality risk? Am J Public Health 1992;82:1105-12.
[228] Rudin-Brown CM, Jenkins RW, Whitehead T, Burns PC. Could ESC (Electronic Stability Control) change the way we drive? Traffic Inj Prev 2009;10(4):10(4):340-7.
[229] Braver ER, Scerbo M, Kufera JA, Alexander MT, Volpini K, Lloyd JP. Deaths among drivers and right-front passengers in frontal collisions: redesigned air bags relative to first-generation air bags. Traffic Inj Prev 2008;9(1):48-58.
[230] Liu BC, Ivers R, Norton R, Boufous S, Blows S, Lo SK. Helmets for preventing injury in motorcycle riders. Cochrane Database Syst Rev 2008;1:CD004333. doi: 10.1002/14651858. CD004333.pub3.
[231] Ludvigsson JF, Stiris T, Del Torso S, Mercier JC, Valiulis A, Hedjipanayis A. European Academy of Paediatrics statement: Vison zero for child deaths in traffic accidents. Eur J Pediatr 2017 Jan 7. doi: 10.1007/s00431-016-2836-1. [Epub ahead of print].
[232] Kardamanidis K, Martiniuk A, Ivers RQ, Stevenson MR, Thistlethwaite K. Motorcycle rider training for the prevention of road traffic crashes. Cochrane Database Syst Rev 2010;10:CD005240. doi: 10.1002/14651858.CD005240.pub2.
[233] Vernick J, Guohua L, Ogaitis S, et al: Effects of high school driver education on motor vehicle crashes, violations, and licensure. Am J Prev Med 1999;16:40-46.
[234] Brown RC, Gains MJ, Greydanus DE. Driver education: A position paper of the Society for Adolescent Medicine, 1992. URL: http://www.adolescenthealth.org/sa...ies/position/driver_education.html.
[235] Mayhew DR, Simpson HM, Williams AF, Ferguson SA: Effectiveness and role of driver education and training in graduated licensing system. J Public Health Policy 1998;19:51-67.
[236] Campbell BT, Borrup K, Derbyshire M, Rogers S, Lapidus G. Efficacy of driving simulator training for novice teen drivers. Conn Med 2016;80(5):291-6.
[237] Gaines BA, Vitale CA. Teenagers—we thought we knew—we didn't—lessons learned. J Trauma 2009;67(Suppl);S58-61.
[238] Senserrick T, Ivers R, Boufous S, Chen HY, Norton R, Stevenson M et al. Young driver education programs that build resilience have potential to reduce road crashes. Pediatrics 2009;124(5):1287-92.
[239] Laird RD. Parenting adolescent drivers is both a continuation of parenting from earlier periods and an anticipation of a new challenge. Accid Anal Prev 2014;69:5-14.
[240] Brookland R, Begg D, Langley J, Ameratunga S. Parental influence on adolescent compliance with graduated driver licensing conditions and crashes as a restricted licensed driver: New Zealand drivers study. Accid Anal Prev 2014;69:30-9.
[241] Curry AE, Peek-Asa C, Hamann CJ, Mirman JH. Effectiveness of parent-focused interventions to increase teen driver safety: a critical review. J Adolesc Health 2015;57(Suppl 1): S6-14.

[242] Shope JT, Zakrajsek JS, Finch S, Bingham CR, O'Neil J, Yano S, et al. Translation to primary care of an effective teen safe driving program for parents. Clin Pediatr (Phila) 2016;55(11):1026-35.
[243] Sagberg F, Selpi, Piccinini GF, Engström J. A review of research on driving styles and road safety. Hum Factors 2015;57(7):1248-75.
[244] Ehsani JP, Li K, Simons-Morton BG, Fox Tree-McGrath C, Perlus JG, O'Brien F, Klauer SG. Conscientious personality and young drivers' crash risk. J Safety Res 2015;54:83-7.
[245] Bagdadi O, Varhelyi A. Jerky driving-an indicator of accident proneness? Accid Anal Prev 2011;43(4):1359-63.
[246] Ker K, Roberts I, Collier T, Renton F, Bunn F. Post-license driver education for the prevention of road traffic crashes. Cochrane Database Syst Rev 2003;3:CD003734.
[247] Ian R, Irene K. Cochrane Injuries Group Driver Education Reviewers. School based driver education for the prevention of traffic crashes. Cochrane Database Syst Rev 2001;3:CD003201.
[248] Peek-Asa C, Britton C, Young T, Pawlovich M, Falb S. Teenage driver crash incidence and factors influencing crash injury by rurality. J Safety Res 2010;41(6):487-92.
[249] Williams AF: Graduated licensing comes to the United States. Inj Prev 1999;5:133-5.
[250] Williams AF, McCartt AT, Sims LB. History and current status of state graduated driver licensing (GLS) laws in the United States. J Safety Res 2016;56:9-15.
[251] Society for Adolescent Health and Medicine, D'Angelo LJ, Halpern-Felsher BL, Abraham A. Adolescents and driving: a position paper of the Society for Adolescent Health and Medicine. J Adolesc Health 2010;47(2):212-4.
[252] McKnight AJ, Peck RC. Graduated driver licensing: what works? Inj Prev 2002;8(Suppl 2):ii32-6.
[253] Ferguson SA, Teoh ER, McCartt AT. Progress in teenage crash risk during the last decade. J Safety Res 2007;38(2):137-45.
[254] Rajaratnam SM, Landrigan CP, Wang W, Kaprielian R, Moore RT, Czeisler CA. Teen crashes declined after Massachusetts raised penalties for graduated licensing law restricting night driving. Health Aff (Millwood) 2015;34(6):963-70.
[255] Shults RA, Williams AF. Graduated driver licensing night driving restrictions and drivers age 16 or 17 years involved in fatal night crashes-United States, 2009-2014. MMWR 2016;65(29):725-30.
[256] Zhu M, Cummings P, Zhao S, Rice T. The association between graduated driver licensing laws and travel behaviors among adolescents: An analysis of the US National Household Travel Surveys. BMC Public Health 2016;16:647. doi: 10.1186/s12889-016-3206-7.
[257] Cavazos-Rehg PA, Housten AJ, Krauss MJ, Sowles SJ, Spitznagel EL, Chaloupka FJ, et al. Selected state policies and associations with alcohol use behaviors and risky driving behaviors among youth: findings from Monitoring the Future Study. Alcohol Clin Exp Res 2016;40(5):1030-6.
[258] Chen LH, Baker SP, Li G. Graduated driver licensing programs and fatal crashes of 16-year-old drivers: a national evaluation. Pediatrics 2006;118(1):56-62.

[259] Ehsani JP, Bingham CR, Shope JT. The effect of the learner license Graduated Driver Licensing components on teen drivers' crashes. Accid Anal Prev 2013;59:327-36.
[260] McCartt AT, Teoh ER. Tracking progress in teenage driver crash risk in the United States since the advent of graduated driver licensing programs. J Safety Res 2015;53:1-9.
[261] Fell JC, Jones K, Romano E, Voas R. An evaluation of graduated driver licensing effects on fatal crash involvements of young drivers in the United States. Traffic Inj Prev 2011;12(5):423-31.
[262] Hartling L, Wiebe N, Russell K, Petruk J, Spinola C, Klassen TP. Graduated driver licensing for reducing motor vehicle crashes among young drivers. Cochrane Database Syst Rev 2004;2:CD003300.
[263] Russell KF, Vandermeer B, Hartling L. Graduated driver licensing for reducing motor vehicle crashes among young drivers. Cochrane Database Syst Rev 2011;10:CD003300. doi.1002/14651858.CD003300.pub3.
[264] Masten SV, Foss RD, Mashall SW. Graduated driver licensing and fatal crashes involving 16- to 19-year-old drivers. JAMA 2011;306(10):1098-103.
[265] Masten SV, Foss RD, Mashall SW. Graduated driver licensing program component calibrations and their association with fatal crash involvement. Accid Anal Prev 2013;57:105-13.
[266] Mirman JH, Curry AE, Winston FK, Wang W, Elliott MR, Schultheis MT, et al. Effect of the teen driving plan on the driving performance of teenagers before licensure: a randomized clinical trial. JAMA Pediatr 2014;168(8):764-71.
[267] Driving among high school students—United States, 2013. MMWR 2015;64(12):313-7.
[268] Williams AF. Commentary: teenage driver fatal crash rate trends: what do they reveal? Traffic Inj Prev 2014;15(7):663-5.
[269] Shults RA, Banerjee T, Perry T. Who's not driving among U.S. high school seniors: A close look at race/ethnicity, socioeconomic factors, and driving status. Traffic Inj Prev 2016;17(8):803-9.
[270] Chapman EA, Masten SV, Browning KK. Crash and traffic violations before and after licensure for novice California drivers subject to different driver licensing requirements. J Safety Res 2014;50:125-38.
[271] Buckley L, Chapman RL, Sheehan M. Young driver distraction: state of the evidence and directions for behavior change programs. J Adolesc Health 2014;54(Suppl 5):S12-21.
[272] Monroe K, Irons E, Crew M, Norris J, Nichols M, King WD. Trends in Alabama in teen driving death and injury. J Trauma Acute Care Surg 2014;77(3 Suppl 1):S51-4.
[273] Zhu M, Zhao S, Long DL, Curry AE. Association of graduated driver licensing with driver, non-driver, and total fatalities among adolescents. Am J Prev Med 2016;51(1):63-70.
[274] Simons-Morton BG, Klauer SG, Ouimet MC, Guo F, Albert PS, Lee SE, et al. Naturalistic teen driving study: findings and lessons learned. J Safety Res 2015;54:41-4.

[275] Curry AE, Pfeiffer MR, Durbin DR, Elliott MR. Young driver crash rates by licensing age, driving experience, and license phase. Accid Anal Prev 2015;80:243-50.
[276] Gulliver P, Begg D, Brookland R, Ameratunga S, Langley J. Learner driver experiences and crash risk as an unsupervised driver. J Safety Res 2013;46:41-6.
[277] Li K, Simons-Morton BG, Hingson R. Impaired-driving prevalence among US high school students: associations with substance use and risky driving behaviors. Am J Public Health 2013;103(11):e71-7.
[278] McNally B, Bradley GL. Re-conceptualizing the reckless driving behavior of young drivers. Accid Anal Prev 2014;70:245-57.
[279] Freydier C, Berthelon C, Bastien-Toniazzo M, Gineyt G. Divided attention in young drivers under the influence of alcohol. J Safety Res 2014;49:13-8.
[280] Rudisill TM, Zhao S, Abate MA, Coben JH, Zhu M. Trends in drug use among drivers killed in the U.S. traffic crashes, 1999-2010. Accid Anal Prev 2014;70:178-87.
[281] Wilson FA, Stimpson JP, Pagán JA. Fatal crashes from drivers testing positive for drugs in the U.S., 1993-2010. Public Health Rep 2014;129(40):342-50.
[282] Zwerling C, Jones MP: Evaluation of the effectiveness of low blood alcohol concentration laws for younger drivers. Am J Prev Med 1999;16:76-80.
[283] Tsai VW, Anderson CL, Vaca FE. Young female drivers in fatal crashes: recent trends, 1995-2004. Traffic Inj Prev 2008;9(1):65-9.
[284] Scagnolari S, Walker J, Maggi R. Young drivers' night-time mobility preferences and attitude toward alcohol consumption: A hybrid model. Accid Anal Prev 2015;83:74-89.
[285] Piastrelli DA, Srour MK, Salim A, Margulies DR. Attitudes and behaviors on alcohol use and impaired driving in adolescents. J Surg Res 2011;170(1):10-3.
[286] DeJong W, Winsten JA. The use of designated drivers by US college students: A national study. J Am Coll Health 1999;47:151-156.
[287] Coben JH, Larkin GL. Effectiveness of ignition interlock devices in reducing drunk driving recidivism. Am J Prev Med 1999;16(1- S):81-7.
[288] McArthur, D.L, Kraus JF. The specific deterrence of administrative per se laws in reducing drunk driving recidivism. Am J Prev Med 1999;16(1 S):68-75.
[289] Schechtman E, Bar-Gera H, Musicant O. Driver views on speed and enforcement. Accid Anal Prev 2016;89:9-21.
[290] Bates L, Allen S, Watson B. The influence of elements of procedural justice and speed cameras enforcement on young novice driver self-reported speeding. Accid Anal Prev 2016;92:34-42.
[291] Wilson C, Willis C, Hendrikz JK, Bellamy N. Speed enforcement detection devices for preventing road traffic injuries. Cochrane Database Syst Rev 2006;2:CD004607.
[292] Wilson C, Willis C, Hendrikz JK, Le Brocque R, Bellamy N. Speed cameras for the prevention of road traffic injuries and death. Cochrane Database Syst Rev 2010;11:CD004607. doi: 10.1002/14651858.CD004607.pub4.
[293] Sadeghnejad F, Miknami S, Hydarnia A, Montazeri A. Seat-belt use among drivers and front passengers: an observational study from the Islamic Republic of Iran. East Mediterr Health J 2014;20(8):491-7.

[294] Houston M, Cassabaum V, Matzick S, Rapstine, Terry S, Uribe P, et al. Teen traffic safety campaign: competition is the key. J Trauma 2010;68(3):511-4.
[295] Nambisan SS, Vasudevan V. Is seat belt usage by front seat passengers related to seat belt usage by their drivers? J Safety Res 2007;38(5):545-55.
[296] Kidd DG, McCartt AT. Drivers' attitudes toward front or rear child passenger belt use and seat belt reminders at these seating positions. Traffic Inj Prev 2014;15(3):276-86.
[297] Peek-Asa C. The effect of random alcohol screening in reducing motor vehicle crash injuries. Am J Prev Med 1999;16(1S):57-67.
[298] Goss CW, Van Bramer LD, Gilner JA, Porter TR, Roberts IG, Diguiseppi C. Increased police patrols for preventing alcohol-impaired driving. Cochrane Database Syst Rev 2008;4:CD005242. doi: 10.1002/14651858.CD005242.pub2.
[299] Ker K, Chinnock P. Interventions in the alcohol server setting for preventing injuries. Cochrane Database Syst Rev 2008;3:CD005244. doi: 10.1002/14651858.CD005244.pub3.
[300] Hellinga LA, McCartt AT, Haire ER. Choice of teenagers' vehicles and views on vehicle safety: survey of parents of novice teenage drivers. J Safety Res 2007;38(6):707-13.
[301] Wogalter MS, Lim RW, Nyester PG. On the hazard of quiet vehicles to pedestrians and drivers. Appl Ergon 2014;45(5):1306-12.
[302] Hitsogui M, Matsui Y. Safety of the Japanese K-car in a real-world low-severity frontal collision. Traffic Inj Prev 2015;16(1):90-4.
[303] McCartt AT, Tech ER. Type, size and age of vehicles driven by teenage drivers killed in crashes during 2008 to 2012. Inj Prev 2015;21(2):133-6.
[304] Evans L, Frick MC: Mass ratio and relative driver fatality risk in two-vehicle crashes. Accid Anal Prev 1993;25:213-224.
[305] Vrklian BH, Anaby D. What vehicle features are considered important when buying an automobile? An examination of driver preferences by age and gender. J Safety Res 2011;42(1):61-5.
[306] Eichelberger AH, Tech ER, McCartt AT. Vehicle choices for teenage drivers: A national survey of U.S. parents. J Safety Res 2015;55:1-5.
[307] Centers for Disease Control and Prevention (CDC). Drivers aged 16 or 17 years involved in fatal crashes—United States, 2004-2008. MMWR 2010;59(41):1329-34.
[308] Potentially preventable deaths from the five leading causes of death—United States, 2008-2010. MMWR 2014;63(17):369-74.
[309] Romano E, Scherer M, Fell J, Taylor E. A comprehensive examination of U.S. laws enacted to reduced alcohol-related crashes among underage drivers. J Safety Res 2015;55:213-21.
[310] Fell JC, Scherer M, Thomas S, Voas RB. Assessing the impact of twenty underage drinking laws. J Stud Alcohol Drugs 2016;77(2):249-60.
[311] Pressley JC, Addison D, Dawson P, Nelson SS. Graduated driver license complaint teens involved in fatal motor vehicle crashes. J Trauma Acute Care Surg 2015;79(3 Suppl 1):S33-41.
[312] Gillan JS. Legislative advocacy is a key to addressing teen driving deaths. Inj Prev 2006;12(Suppl 1):i44-8.

[313] Scott-Parker B, Senserrick T. A call to improve sampling methodology and reporting in young novice driver research. Inj Pre 2016 Jul 27pii: injuryprev-2016-042105.
[314] Curry AE, Kim KH, Pfeiffer MR. Inaccuracy of Federal Highway Administration's licensed driver data: implications on young driver trends. J Adolesc Health 2014;55(3):452-4.
[315] Nilboer M, Borst JP, van Rijn H, Taatgen NA. Driving and multitasking: the good, the bad, and the dangerous. Front Psychol 2016;7:1718. eCollection 2016.
[316] Chaurand N, Delhomme P. Cyclists and drivers in road interactions: A comparison of perceived crash risk. Accid Anal Prev 2013;50:1176-84.
[317] Sleet DA, Ballesteros MF, Borse NN. A review of unintentional injuries in adolescents. Annu Rev Public Health 2010;31:195-212.
[318] Announcement. Recommendation regarding universal motorcycle helmet laws—Community Prevention Services Task Force. WWMR 2014;63(25):554.
[319] Audrey S, Langford R. Dying to get out: young drivers, safety and social inequity. Inj Prev 2014;20(1):1-6.
[320] O'Connor SS, Shain LM, Whitehill JM, Ebel BE. Measuring a conceptual model of the relationship between compulsive cell phone use in-vehicle cell use and motor vehicle crash. Accid Anal Prev 2017;99(Pt A):372-8.

In: Children and Youth
Editors: Donald E. Greydanus et al.

ISBN: 978-1-53611-102-6
© 2017 Nova Science Publishers, Inc.

Chapter 3

DEMOGRAPHICS

Kathryn White[*], *MA*

Department of Pediatric and Adolescent Medicine,
Western Michigan University Homer Stryker MD School of Medicine,
Kalamazoo, Michigan, US

There has been a significant decrease in traffic injuries and fatalities in the last decade due to major advances in restraint systems in vehicles and by large initiatives that have taken place to educate parents, children and adolescents on the importance of safety in and around cars. However, motor vehicle related crashes continue to be the leading cause of death and injury for children ages 5-19 years. There are a number of different motor vehicle related crashes that a child or adolescent can be involved in; occupant of a vehicle, pedestrian and pedal cyclist. As a result, children and adolescents are exposed to a variety of injuries and psychological stress from these encounters. The following chapter will provide demographic data related to children and adolescents involvement in these different types of crashes along with the various physical injuries and nonphysical injuries that can occur as a result. This will signify the importance of and demonstrate how often this age group is and can be affected by traffic crashes and the impending trauma that is likely occurring, even in the absence of physical injury.

---

[*] Correspondence: Kathryn White, MA, Temporary Limited Licensed Psychologist, Department of Pediatric and Adolescent Medicine, Western Michigan University Homer Stryker MD School of Medicine, 1000 Oakland Drive, Kalamazoo, MI 49008, United States. Email: kathryn.white@med.wmich.edu.

INTRODUCTION

Staggering statistics reveal that motor vehicle crashes are the leading cause of death and disability in children over the age of 1 year (1). Organizations began studying this phenomenon in the late 1970s and have dedicated numerous resources to reduce these statistics (2). From 1978-1991 the rate of fatalities decreased by 24% for children under the age of 19 years, but remained stagnant thereafter (1). It was suggested that these statistics did not improve for several possibilities; limited restraint system designs, the misuse or nonuse of restraint systems and because of an increase need to travel (1). This prompted a demand for further data to address this issue.

In the late 1990s a comprehensive investigation was conducted by the "Partners for Child Passenger Safety" to determine how and why children and adolescents were killed or injured in crashes (2). The results of these studies began a multi-tiered initiative. The past decade has involved the nations drive to educate parents, children, and adolescents on the importance of safety in and around cars with particular attention towards the appropriate use of restraints (i.e., car seats, booster seats, seatbelts and helmets). Overall, this campaign has been a successful endeavor.

According to the National Highway Traffic Safety Administration (NHTSA) the number of children (aged 14 years or younger) killed in a motor vehicle or traffic related crash is down 45% from 2005 to 2013 with injuries down 28% from 2005 to 2013 (3). Although these statistics are promising, the Center for Disease Control (CDC) continues to report that injuries sustained in a motor vehicle or traffic related crash remain the leading cause of death for children ages 5-19 years and are the cause of a large number of children being treated in an emergency department each hour (4).

These statistics highlight the degree to which a child or adolescent is likely to be involved in a motor vehicle or traffic related crash before they reach adulthood which in turn has the potential to expose them to any number of physical and/or mental health related injuries which further supports the need for immediate intervention to reduce lingering effects.

CHILDREN AND ADOLESCENTS

According to a report completed by NHTSA there were 61 million children (14 years and younger) in the United States making up 19 percent of the population in 2014 (3). In addition, there were over 10 million police reported crashes in that same year (5). These crashes resulted in 32,675 fatalities with 1,070 of them involving children (3). Of the 1,070 child fatalities, 774 were occupants in a vehicle and 296 were either pedestrians, pedal cyclists or other (3).

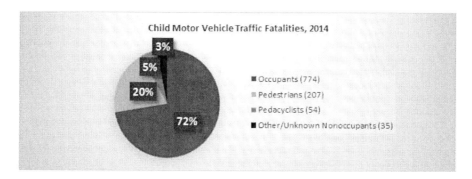

Figure 1. Source: 2014 NHTSA Traffic Safety Facts; Children (3)

The 10 million crashes that occurred overall in 2014 caused an estimated 167,000 children to be injured (3). These statistics indicate that on average 3 children are killed and 458 are injured every day in traffic related crashes (3). It is also estimated that 55% of the children killed and 50% that were injured in a crash were male (3).

These statistics confirm that a large number of children are exposed to traffic related crashes and therefore trauma as well. However, a child does not simply have to be injured in order to experience trauma related symptoms or to be directly affected by this type of incident. In 2014 there were an estimated 10 million crashes, and, although upsetting, only 167,000 children out of these 10 million crashes were injured. This brings to light a large number of children who are not being physically injured, which is estimated to be around 690,000 children, but are exposed none the less (6).

Uninjured children can suffer "injuries" and psychological stress merely by their exposure to a traffic crash either by witnessing others who were injured or deceased as a result of a traffic related crash or simply by the crash itself. Further, there were over 30,000 fatalities not involving children, which makes it safe to assume that children are directly affected by these losses as well which further exposes them to a trauma.

Adolescents

A 2014 report completed by NHTSA indicated there were 214.1 million licensed drivers in the United States and of those 11.7 million were young drivers age 15-20 (5). Young drivers are defined as those that are in operation of the vehicle at the time of a crash (5). Reported statistics indicate that of the 11.7 million young drivers in 2014, over one million of them were the driver in a police reported crash (5). Of these one million crashes 1,717 young drivers were killed and an estimated 170,000 were injured that same year (5). In addition, in 2014 743 children and adolescents under the age of 20 were passengers whom died as a result of a crash involving a young driver (5).

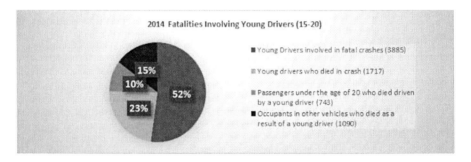

Figure 2. Source: NHTSA 2014 Traffic Safety Facts; Young Drivers (5)

Statistics indicate that in 2014 males were 2.3 times more likely to be involved in a fatal motor vehicle crash than females and 26% of the young drivers were intoxicated at the time of the crash (5). In 2014 285 (10%) of adolescents (aged 15-19) were the distracted driver involved in a fatal crash and 230 (9%) were killed as a result of a distracted related crash (7).

This data, like the data for children, indicates that young drivers and adolescents have the potential to be dramatically impacted either by loss of life, injury or psychological stress due to their involvement in traffic related incidents in their teens. In addition, because they are now the drivers of the vehicles their role and level of responsibility increases which can directly impact their response to a trauma of a crash they are involved in.

MOTOR VEHICLE AND TRAFFIC RELATED CRASHES

Many terms are used to describe what the general public typically refer to as a car accident. The World Health Organization and the CDC (Center for Disease Control and Prevention) uses the term road traffic injury, the US Census Bureau uses the term motor vehicle accidents, some law enforcement departments further distinguish by using the term personal injury or property damage crashes, while the National Highway Traffic Safety Administration (NHTSA) uses the term motor vehicle traffic crashes.

Around the late 1990's a campaign was created by NHTSA to change the way people view traffic related crashes with a push to change terminology from an accident to a crash. An "accident" signifies that the event was outside of human influence or control and therefore unavoidable, which in turn worked against conveying the need for resources to combat the significant problem of motor vehicle collisions (8). The goal was to change the focus to finding ways to prevent these crashes and the injuries that occur because of them (8). This initiative began around the time that the "Partners for Child Passenger Safety" began their comprehensive investigation into the impact of crashes on children and adolescents which in turn created the large initiative to find ways to reduce injury and death for this population and the population as a whole.

Regardless of the terminology used, statistics have proven that injuries sustained because of crashes are significant for the welfare of children and adolescents across the nation. There are several ways a child or adolescent can be involved in a motor vehicle or traffic related crash. The most common is as an occupant in a vehicle while others include as a pedestrian or a pedal cyclists injured by a motor vehicle. All of which can result in substantial physical or mental health related injuries.

OCCUPANT IN A VEHICLE

A vehicle traffic crash is defined as "an incident that involved one or more vehicles where at least one vehicle was in transport and the crash originated on a public traffic way, such as a road or highway and exclude those that occur on private property (i.e., parking lots and driveways)" (3). Being an occupant in a vehicle differs from a child to adolescent. Children under the age of 15 are generally considered the passenger, while those over 15 can either be a passenger or a driver. As reported, children and adolescents are injured and killed more often as an occupant of a vehicle then in any other traffic related crash, likely because the last couple of decades have shown an increase in people owning and driving vehicles (9).

Children

Children, especially young children, are often reliant on the driver or older occupant to ensure they are properly restrained. Estimates indicate that when a driver is unrestrained 70% of children are also unrestrained (3). Drivers are the role models for the younger generation and can impact the child's future use of restraints once they become young drivers which in turn impacts the new generation of occupants.

Statistics have reported that with the movement to educate the population of the importance of various restraints and with cars taking the initiative to develop safety features, like air bags, the number of injuries and deaths have significantly declined. It is estimated that in 2014 252 children under the age of 4 were saved because of the use of child restraints, with 236 of these due to the use of child safety seats and 17 because of seatbelts (3). It is suggested that if the use of child restraints were at 100% an additional 37 children could have been saved (3).

Adolescents

Young drivers are three times more likely to be involved in a traffic crash than adults (10). There are several reasons that have been identified for this which include; inadequate observation experience, use of technology in the vehicle (cell phones), distractions by peer passengers, night driving and risky behavior (10,11). Research has also determined that summer is a particularly dangerous time for young drivers and account for 7 of the 10 deadliest days for them (11). Young drivers and the use of restraints also have a direct correlation with alcohol consumption with a decrease in use being directly affected by the increase in use of alcohol (5). Statistics further report that an estimated 12,802 people 5 and older were saved due to the use of seat belts, 2,396 people 13 and older due to frontal air bags and 1,669 due to the use of motorcycle helmets (12).

For adolescents, nationwide measures have been taken in an attempt to try and reduce the statistics regarding crashes involving young drivers with the development of several interventions. For example, the production of the graduated driver license policy, initiatives that focus on educating young drivers on the risk of the growing problem of distracted driving and alcohol awareness. One such organization is the Center for Injury Research and Prevention through the Children's Hospital of Philadelphia which is focused on reducing the frequency and severity of young drivers cashes, injuries and fatalities (13). Their research and interventions have led them to three areas of focus; improving and acquiring teens skills through training, compliance with the Graduated License provisions and improving their behaviors while driving (13).

These statistics are encouraging for both children and adolescents and the resources that have been developed over the last decade have proved to be very beneficial, however the statistics also signify that traffic related crashes continue to be a significant source of trauma among this population.

PEDESTRIAN INVOLVED CRASHES

Stories are reported across the nation of pedestrian involved car crashes. The saddest of which are those involving children and adolescents. A pedestrian is any person on foot, walking, running, jogging, hiking, sitting or lying down, who are involved in motor vehicle traffic crash (3). An overarching number of crashes that occur involving pedestrians are due primarily to the fault of the pedestrian (9).

Children

Studies have determined that children are one of the age groups that are most vulnerable to being involved in a pedestrian car crash (9). Statistics indicate that nearly 8,000 children under the age of 14 are injured a year with 5,000 of them being boys in pedestrian traffic related crashes (3). Child pedestrian accidents typically occur by a single-vehicle, in urban areas at a non-intersection location during daylight hours (161 in 2014), but in 2014, 4 were due to multiple vehicles (3).

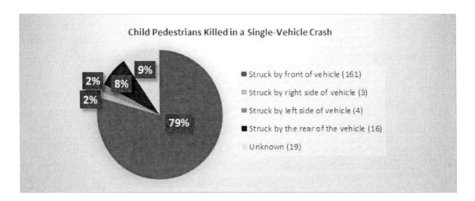

Figure 3. Source: NHTSA 2014 Traffic Safety Fact Sheet; Children (3)

Adolescent

Statistics indicate that in 2010 there were 413 pedestrians between the ages of 10-20 years killed in a traffic related crash (11). Several factors are associated with a higher likelihood of being at risk and include; being male, living in an urban area, walking initiatives try and make adolescents aware of the risk of texting and walking. Studies have found that those that text and walk took about two seconds longer to cross a street then those who were not texting (11).

PEDAL CYCLIST INVOLVED CRASHES

Pedal cyclists are riders of bicycles (two-wheel, non-motorized cycles) and other cycles (tricycles and unicycles) powered solely by pedals who are involved in motor vehicle traffic crashes (3). Like pedestrian related crashes, pedal cyclist's crashes are mostly caused by human error (14).

Children and adolescents

726 pedal cyclists were killed in 2014, with 54 being children under the age of 14 years (3). Further an estimated 50,000 people were injured with 6,000 of those being children (3).

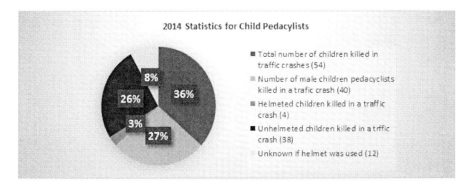

Figure 4. Source: NHTSA 2014 Traffic Safety Fact Sheet; Children (3).

As children get older and become young drivers their use of bicycles may decrease however their risk of involvement in these types of crashes do not necessarily decline since now they are on the other side as the driver. Studies from around the world have determined that often children that are injured in bicycle crashes are more likely a result of doing tricks, riding too fast, or losing control while teenagers are more due to collisions with a motor vehicle (14). Most causative factor regarding injuries and fatalities by a motor vehicles are due to failing to look properly (by either driver or rider), while another factor includes the rider entering the road from the pavement (14).

The research and studies that have looked into why children and adolescents are involved in these types of crashes have also begun campaigns to reduce the statistics. The most noteworthy is the push for the use of helmets. Many organizations, like Safe Kids, have programs that encourage their use and proper fit. With this push, statistics indicate that it reduces head injuries related to a crash by 50% (15).

TYPES OF INJURIES

As stated previously, traffic related crashes are the most common way a child or adolescent obtains injuries. There are several types of "injuries" a child or adolescent can sustain when involved in these incidents. Most commonly thought of are physical injuries; bumps, bruises, breaks etcetera that are easily seen or felt. However, being an occupant of a vehicle, a pedal cyclist or a pedestrian involved in a traffic related crash is also the most common traumatic event that a child will be involved in during their childhood (16). Therefore, even more probable are those "injuries" that are not visible and cause psychological stress. These are likely more common because they not only affect those that are injured, but also those that are not-injured and those that are simply exposed either directly or indirectly to these events.

Physical injuries

When thinking about a traffic related crash and the consequences of being involved in such an incident we commonly think about the physical injuries that one may obtain. Seriousness of injuries sustained when a child or adolescent involved in a motor vehicle or traffic related crash can be affected by many different factors such as the seriousness of the crash, use/misuse or nonuse of restraint systems, speed, and location of impact. Further, types of injuries can also vary greatly and can range from minor bumps and bruises to traumatic brain injuries and death. Studies have revealed that children who sustain injuries during a crash can have a worse outcome than similar injuries sustained by adults (17).

This is most concerning when it comes to children who suffer from head trauma. Since children are in a continual path of development, effects from injuries may not become observable until an expectant milestone is not reached (17). Examples include frontal lobe damage that may not become apparent until adolescence when higher level reasoning is expected or when a child enters school and begins to show signs of learning disorders that may be a result of a previous head trauma (17). When a child or adolescent is injured, their injuries are often quickly treated and monitored by physicians, because they are recognizable and diagnosable. Traffic crashes are the leading cause of injuries in this population and therefore are also the most likely to be experienced.

Psychological injuries

Prior to 2002 there have been a limited number of studies that have documented the effects of trauma on children (16). As previously stated traffic related crashes are not only the leading cause of injuries and death for children and adolescents but are also the leading cause of trauma for this population. When children and adolescents experience a trauma they can react and experience psychological effects in a variety of ways which largely go unnoticed or treated. Psychological effects of exposure can be experienced by the development of an anxiety, depressive or trauma and stressor related disorder or a combination of them.

When a child or adolescent is injured in a crash they are often immediately treated by or in contact with a physician. At that time a physician who has been trained to screen for trauma symptoms, can determine if a child has any signs related to their exposure. Children will likely present with a few symptoms initially (16). When injuries require further follow up, trauma symptoms can and should be monitored and assessed for by their pediatrician, since trauma symptoms can also be delayed. If a child does not require a follow-up or if they have not initially expressed trauma symptoms, later reactions may go unnoticed or untreated.

Even more concerning is the hundreds of thousands of children and adolescents who experience psychological stress even when they do not sustain injuries as a results of a crash, are not directly involved in the crash but are exposed because of the loss of or injury sustained to a family member or simply by witnessing a crash. Trauma related diagnoses, specifically post-traumatic stress disorder and acute stress disorder account for direct and indirect exposure (18), which makes the propensity for such trauma even more likely.

The complexity of mental health diagnoses can be a difficult area for physicians, who are generally the first to encounter individuals involved in these incidents, to navigate especially with this population. Often children and adolescents have a poor insight and a limited ability to recognize and express feelings associated with a mental health diagnosis than they have when they are hurt physically. In addition, because psychological disorders have varying symptoms associated with them and can be delayed, invisible, difficult to express or understand can further result in them being misinterpreted (as a behavior problem in children) or not recognized at all. Psychological disorders are therefore easily overlooked because of the absence of visible wounds, which makes it likely that they are more prevalent when all exposures are taken into account.

Conclusion

Promising statistics regarding the number of children and adolescents being injured or killed in the past decade have been reported. However, with the increasing need to drive and unlikeliness that car crashes will become extinct, and since it continues to be the leading cause of injury and death, the impact they will have on children and adolescents needs to be an area that is addressed further.

In particular, the psychological stress that these incidents cause is of specific importance. It was only recently that traffic crashes were highlighted as a preventable act which in turn encouraged research and initiatives to be developed in order to wage war against the troubling statistics. The results have been encouraging and many lives have been saved, however, a problem continues. In addition, minimal research about the effects that these crashes have on children and adolescents, especially those that are not physically injured, has not been done.

The statistics presented in this review emphasize the exposure that children and adolescents have to traffic related crashes either by being injured or being directly or indirectly involved. Trauma's that occur in this population can carry over into adulthood and affect many facets of life. Research regarding this impact would likely produce results that would encourage early detection and treatment in order to reduce future affects that these traumas could have on this population.

REFERENCES

[1]   Partners for Child Passenger Safety, 2000. URL: https://injury.research.chop.edu/sites/default/files/documents/int_reprt_00.pdf.
[2]   Durbin DR, Bhatia E, Holmes JH, Shaw KN, Werner JV, Sorenson W, et al. Partners for child passenger safety: A unique child-specific crash surveillance system. Accid Anal Prev 2001;33(3):407–12.
[3]   Children date, 2014. National Highway Traffic Safety Administration, National Center for Statistics and Analysis, 2016. URL: http://www-nrd.nhtsa.dot.gov/Pubs/811620.pdf%5Cnhttp://www-nrd.nhtsa.dot.gov/Pubs/809778.pdf.
[4]   Road Traffic Safety. Child Safety and Injury Prevention, CDC Injury Center. URL: https://www.cdc.gov/safechild/Road_Traffic_Injuries/index.html
[5]   Young driver's data, 2014. National Highway Traffic Safety Administration, National Center for Statistics and Analysis, 2016. URL: https://crashstats.nhtsa.dot.gov/Api/Public/ViewPublication/812278.
[6]   Romano E, Kelley-Baker T. Child passengers injured in motor vehicle crashes. J Safety Res 2015; 52:1–8.
[7]   Teens and distracted driving data. National Highway Traffic Safety Administration National Center for Statistics and Analysis, 2016. URL: https://crashstats.nhtsa.dot.gov/Api/Public/ViewPublication/812253.
[8]   Anikeeff P. Crashes aren't accident campaign, 1997. URL: http://web.archive.org/web/20040409081644/http://www.nhtsa.dot.gov/nhtsa/announce/NhtsaNow/Archive/1997/v3.11/.

[9] Lee C, Abdel-Aty M. Comprehensive analysis of vehicle-pedestrian crashes at intersections in Florida. Accid Anal Prev 2005;37(4):775–86.
[10] McDonald CC, Curry AE, Kandadai V, Sommers MS, Winston FK. Comparison of teen and adult driver crash scenarios in a nationally representative sample of serious crashes. Accid Anal Prev 2014;72:302–8. doi.org/10.1016/j.aap.2014.07.016.
[11] The Office of Adolescent Health, 2013. URL: https://www.hhs.gov/ash/oah/news/e-updates/eupdate-july2013.html.
[12] Quick facts 2014. National Highway Traffic Safety Administration National Center for Statistics and Analysis, 2016. URL: https://crashstats.nhtsa.dot.gov/Api/Public/ViewPublication/812234.
[13] Teen driver safety. Center for Injury Research and Prevention. URL: https://injury.research.chop.edu/traffic-injury-prevention/teen-driver-safety#.WGvFVk2FPIU.
[14] The Royal Society for the Prevention of Accidents. Cycling accidents facts and figures: August 2014. URL: http://www.rospa.com/road-safety/advice/pedal-cyclists/facts-figures/
[15] Fatality facts, 2015. Insurance Institute for Highway Safety Highway Loss Data Institute, 2016. URL: http://www.iihs.org/iihs/topics/t/pedestrians-and-bicyclists/fatalityfacts/bicycles/2014.
[16] Winston FK, Kassam-adams N, Neill CV, Ford J, Newman E, Baxt C, et al. After pediatric traffic injury. Pediatrics 2011;109(6): URL: http://www.pediatrics.org/cgi/content/full/109/6/e90.
[17] National Highway Traffic Safety Administration (NHTSA). Children injured in motor vehicle traffic crashes. Traffic Saf 2010; URL: https://crashstats.nhtsa.dot.gov/Api/Public/ViewPublication/81132518. American Psychiatric Association. DSM-V. Diagnostic and statistical manual of mental disorders, 5th ed. Arlington, VA: APA, 2013.

In: Children and Youth
Editors: Donald E. Greydanus et al.
ISBN: 978-1-53611-102-6
© 2017 Nova Science Publishers, Inc.

Chapter 4

ASSESSMENT OF POSTTRAUMATIC STRESS DISORDER IN CHILDREN AND ADOLESCENTS SUBSEQUENT TO MOTOR VEHICLE CRASH

Kathryn White[*], MA
Department of Pediatric and Adolescent Medicine, Western Michigan University Homer Stryker MD School of Medicine, Kalamazoo, Michigan, US

Statistics regarding the prevalence of motor vehicle and traffic related crashes make it very likely that a child or adolescent will encounter one in their lifetime. Although not all crashes result in an injury or are traumatic, the potential is there. Traumatic experiences can affect individuals in different ways. Some may be resilient and not experience any effects while others may develop symptoms that could qualify for a mental health diagnosis like an anxiety, depressive or trauma or stressor related disorder. One of the more significant responses to a traumatic event is a diagnosis of post-traumatic stress disorder (PTSD). However, in order to meet this diagnosis a significant amount of criteria must be met and others ruled out. Because of this a thorough assessment process that is multifaceted is needed to determine if the data elicits a PTSD

---

[*] Correspondence: Kathryn White, MA, Temporary Limited Licensed Psychologist, Department of Pediatric and Adolescent Medicine, Western Michigan University Homer Stryker MD School of Medicine, 1000 Oakland Drive, Kalamazoo, MI 49008, United States. Email: kathryn.white@med.wmich.edu.

diagnosis, a differential diagnosis or comorbid diagnosis all of which can be used to develop an appropriate treatment plan.

INTRODUCTION

The Center for Disease Control and Prevention (CDC) reports that injuries sustained in a motor vehicle or traffic related crash remains the leading cause of death for children ages 5-19 and are the cause of a large number of children being treated in an emergency department each hour (1). In 2014 there were over 10 million police reported crashes (2). Of those 10 million, 690,000 children were exposed absent a physical injury while 167,000 children were injured (3, 4). Lacking from this statistics are children who experience a traffic related crash indirectly by either witnessing a crash or through the loss of or injury to a family member. These implications highlight the degree to which a child or adolescent is likely to be involved, witness or experience a crash or the consequences of a crash and therefore be subjected to any number of physical injuries or psychological disorders.

Psychological disorders are often easily overlooked, because of the absence of visible wounds. They are also more prevalent than physical injuries because physical injuries require actual involvement in the traffic related crash, where a psychological injury can occur from either witnessing a crash without actual involvement, having a close family member be involved in a crash, or by being a non-injured party to a crash. Trauma related diagnoses, specifically post-traumatic stress disorder and acute stress disorder account for direct and indirect exposure (5), which makes the propensity for a child to experience such trauma even more possible.

Further, when a child experiences a trauma, they can react and experience psychological effects in a variety of ways and can develop an array of disorders like an anxiety, depressive or trauma and stressor related disorder or a combination of them. For the purposes of this chapter the focus will be on how to assess for children and adolescents who may suffer from a post-traumatic stress disorder (PTSD) after exposure to a motor or traffic related crash.

POST-TRAUMATIC STRESS DISORDER DIAGNOSIS

The American Psychological Association defines trauma as "an emotional response to a terrible event" (6). A person's emotional response to these events can produce psychological distress. The "Diagnostic and statistical manual of mental disorders" 5th edition (DSM-5) recognizes that a person's response to a psychological stress is not always clearly defined (5). A person can develop an array of symptoms (i.e., anxiety or fear based) and ways of expression (i.e., aggressive or dissociative) following an exposure (5). One of the trauma related disorders that a person can acquire after an exposure to a traumatic event is post-traumatic stress disorder.

A post-traumatic stress disorder diagnosis is dependent on a person's development of characteristic symptoms following the trauma exposure (5). The DSM-5 clearly outlines the criteria needed for a professional to formally diagnose a patient with PTSD. In addition, it takes into account differences in response dependent on age and has therefore divided the criteria for PTSD into sections for children under the age of 6 years and children older than 6 years. Tables 1, 2 and 3 identify the DSM-5's diagnostic criteria for PTSD.

The DSM-5 was recently released in 2013 with some changes in their language of the PTSD criteria compared to the DSM-IV. Most notably is the language in criterion A, which has enhanced the definition of what constitutes a traumatic event (7). For the purposes of this review, one of the significant changes to the DSM-5 allows for a child to meet qualifications if they learn about a family or close friend's involvement in a serious accident (7). The allowance of direct and indirect exposure does however require some specifications on how the event was experienced (7) and the DSM-5 has tightened criteria A of "learning about" a trauma exposure to only violent or accidental death (8, p. 41).

Screening for post-traumatic stress disorder

As Tables 1, 2 and 3 outline, in order for a person to qualify for a PTSD diagnosis they must meet certain criteria that is representative of this disorder. In addition the person must meet the criteria for longer than a month (5).

Table 1. DSM-5 Criteria for posttraumatic stress disorder diagnostic criteria*

	Diagnostic Criteria
A) Exposure to actual or threatened death, serious injury, or sexual violence in **one (or more)** of the following ways:	1) Directly experiencing the traumatic events 2) Witnessing, in person, the event(s) as it occurred to others 3) Learning that the traumatic event(s) occurred to a close family member or close friend. In cases of actual or threatened death of a family member or friend, the event(s) must have been violent or accidental. 4) Experiencing repeated or extreme exposure to aversive details of the traumatic event(s) (e.g., first responders collecting human remains; police officers repeatedly exposed to details of child abuse). **Note:** Criterion A4 does not apply to exposure through electronic media, television, movies, or pictures, unless this exposure is work related.
B) Presence of **one (or more)** of the following intrusion symptoms associated with the traumatic event(s), beginning after the traumatic event.	1) Recurrent, involuntary, and intrusive distressing memories of the traumatic event(s) **Note:** In children older than 6 years, repetitive play may occur in which themes or aspects of the traumatic event(s) are expressed 2) Recurrent distressing dreams in which the content and/or affect of the dream are related to the traumatic event(s) **Note:** In children, there may be frightening dreams without recognizable content 3) Dissociative reactions (e.g., flashbacks) in which the individual feels or acts as if the traumatic event(s) were recurring. Such reactions may occur on a continuum, with the most extreme expression being a complete loss of awareness of present surroundings **Note:** In children, trauma-specific reenactment may occur in play. 4) Intense or prolonged psychological distress at exposure to internal or external cues that symbolize or resemble an aspect of the traumatic event(s). 5) Marked physiological reactions to internal or external cues that symbolize or resemble an aspect of the traumatic event(s).

Diagnostic Criteria

C) Persistent avoidance of stimuli associated with the traumatic event(s), beginning after the traumatic event(s) occurred, as evidenced by **one or both** of the following:	1) Avoidance of or efforts to avoid distressing memories, thoughts, or feelings about or closely associated with the traumatic event(s). 2) Avoidance of or efforts to avoid external reminders (people, places, conversations, activities, objects, situations) that arouse distressing memories, thoughts, or feelings about or closely associated with the traumatic event(s).
D) Negative alternations in cognitions and mood associated with the traumatic event(s) beginning or worsening after the traumatic event(s) occurred, as evidenced by **two (or more)** of the following:	1) Inability to remember an important aspect of the traumatic event(s) (typically due to dissociative amnesia and not to other factors such as head injury, alcohol, or drugs). 2) Persistent and exaggerated negative beliefs or expectations about oneself, others, or the world (e.g., "I am bad," "No one can be trusted," "The world is completely dangerous," "My whole nervous system is permanently ruined.") 3) Persistent, distorted cognitions about the cause or consequences of the traumatic event(s) that lead the individual to blame himself/herself or others. 4) Persistent negative emotional state (e.g., fear, horror, anger, guilt, or shame). 5) Markedly diminished interest or participation in significant activities. 6) Feelings of detachment or estrangement from others. 7) Persistent inability to experience positive emotions (e.g., inability to experience happiness, satisfaction or loving feelings.)
E) Marked alterations in arousal and reactivity associated with the traumatic event(s), beginning or worsening after the traumatic event(s) occurred, as evidenced by **two (or more)** of the following:	1) Irritable behavior and angry outbursts (with little or no provocation) typically expressed as verbal or physical aggression toward people or objects. 2) Reckless or self-destructive behavior. 3) Hypervigilance 4) Exaggerated startle response 5) Problems with concentration 6) Sleep disturbance (e.g., difficulty falling or staying asleep or restless sleep.)

Table 1. (Continued)

Diagnostic Criteria
F) Duration of the disturbance (Criteria B, C, D, and E) is more than 1 month. G) The disturbance causes clinically significant distress or impairment in social, occupational, or other important areas of functioning. H) The disturbance is not attributable to the physiological effects of a substance (e.g., medication, alcohol) or other medical condition.

* Adapted from the "Diagnostic and Statistical Manual of Mental Disorders, Fifth Edition", by the American Psychiatric Association, Copyright 2013. Pages 271-272 (5).

Note: The following criteria apply to adults, adolescents, and children older than 6 years.

Table 2. DSM-5 Criteria for posttraumatic stress disorder diagnostic criteria*

	Diagnostic Criteria
A) In children 6 and younger exposure to actual or threatened death, serious injury, or sexual violence in **one (or more)** of the following ways:	1) Directly experiencing the traumatic events 2) Witnessing, in person, the event(s) as it occurred to others, especially primary caregivers **Note**: Witnessing does not include events that are witnessed only in electronic media, television, movies, or pictures 3) Learning that the traumatic event(s) occurred to a parent or caregiver.
B) Presence of **one (or more)** of the following intrusion symptoms associated with the traumatic event(s), beginning after the traumatic event.	1) Recurrent, involuntary, and intrusive distressing memories of the traumatic event(s) **Note**: Spontaneous and intrusive memories may not necessarily appear distressing and may be expressed as play reenactment. 2) Recurrent distressing dreams in which the content and/or affect of the dream are related to the traumatic event(s) **Note**: It may not be possible to ascertain that the frightening content is related to the traumatic event. 3) Dissociative reactions (e.g., flashbacks) in which the child feels or acts as if the traumatic event(s) were recurring. (Such reactions may occur on a continuum, with the most extreme expression being a complete loss of awareness of present surroundings.) Such trauma-specific reenactment may occur in play. 4) Intense or prolonged psychological distress at exposure to internal or external cues that symbolize or resemble an aspect of the traumatic event(s). 5) Marked physiological reactions to reminders of the traumatic event(s).

Table 2. (Continued)

	Diagnostic Criteria
D) Alterations in arousal and reactivity associated with the traumatic event(s), beginning or worsening after the traumatic event(s) occurred, as evidenced by **two (or more)** of the following:	1) Irritable behavior and angry outbursts (with little or no provocation) typically expressed as verbal or physical aggression toward people or objects (including extreme temper tantrums.) 2) Hypervigilance 3) Exaggerated startle response 4) Problems with concentration 5) Sleep disturbance (e.g., difficulty falling or staying asleep or restless sleep.)
E) Duration of the disturbance is more than 1 month. F) The disturbance causes clinically significant distress or impairment in relationships with parents, siblings, peers, or other caregivers or with school behavior. G) The disturbance is not attributable to the physiological effects of a substance (e.g., medication, alcohol) or other medical conditions	

* Adapted from the "Diagnostic and Statistical Manual of Mental Disorders, Fifth Edition", by the American Psychiatric Association, Copyright 2013. Pages 272-274 (5).

Note: The following criteria apply to children 6 years and younger.

Table 3. DSM -5 Specifiers for posttraumatic stress disorder*

For both individuals over and under the age of 6 a PTSD diagnosis can have the following specifiers:

Specify whether:
With dissociative symptoms: The individual's symptoms meet the criteria for post-traumatic stress disorder, and in addition, in response to the stressor, the individual experiences persistent or recurrent symptoms of either of the following:

1) **Depersonalization**: Persistent or recurrent experiences of feeling detached from and as if one were an outside observer of, one's mental processes or body (e.g. feeling as though one were in a dream; feeling a sense of unreality of self or body or of time moving slowly).

2) **Derealization**: Persistent or recurrent experience of unreality or surroundings (e.g. the world around the individual is experienced as unreal, dreamlike, distant, or distorted.)

Note: To use this subtype, the dissociative symptoms must not be attributable to the physiological effects of a substance (e.g., blackouts, behavior during alcohol intoxication) or another medical condition (e.g., complex or partial seizures.

Specify with:
With delayed expression: If the full diagnostic criteria are not met until at least 6 months after the event (although the onset and expression of some symptoms may be immediate).

---

* Adapted from the "Diagnostic and Statistical Manual of Mental Disorders, Fifth Edition", by the American Psychiatric Association, Copyright 2013. Pages 272 (5).

As reported previously, a person's reaction to trauma can vary from person to person, therefore the criteria for this disorder encompasses varying forms of responses. While psychological distress following a trauma can be complicated, it can be even more complex when we encounter children. This is because this population is in a continual progression of change in many facets of development which can directly affect their response to a trauma as compared to adults whose development has plateaued. In addition children may have poor insight into their emotions and behaviors, therefore may be unable to relay how the trauma they experienced has impacted them to an evaluator. With this in mind a strong assessment process is needed in order to properly make this diagnosis.

The assessment process for PTSD should be conducted by a professional that is properly trained to evaluate and diagnosis mental health disorders. The method should be multifaceted and contain, but is not limited to, the following; a structured clinical interview that includes both the parents and child, screening assessments along with information obtained from other resources. Whether a PTSD diagnosis is or is not made, obtaining this level of data will allow the evaluator a significant amount of information to articulate their conclusions. In addition, this information can be beneficial in determining what course of treatment should be obtained following the evaluation along with any differential or comorbid diagnoses.

Structured clinical interview

Clinical interviews for children involves "face to face interaction between the interviewer and the interviewee to gather information about a person's behavioral, social, and emotional functioning" (9). Clinical interviews are a symbol of a thorough assessment and are commonly used (9). In particular they are a good way to obtain data from multiple perspectives, and are a great way to establish rapport (9). Although the information that a clinical interview provides is often abundant, obtaining data from multiple sources is strongly recommended before arriving at a diagnosis. This is particularly important when considering a diagnosis of PTSD. In order to formally diagnose this disorder it is important to determine that the symptoms being presented are a direct result of a trauma and not for other reasons (5).

Conducting a structured clinical interview

A structured clinical interview will likely occur during an initial meeting with a family. The purpose of this interview is to obtain a broad range of information which can then lead a clinician to determine what assessments and possible treatments would be appropriate for the patient and possibly the family. These interviews should cover a wide range of areas in order to obtain the most information and can include but is not limited to the following topics;

reason for appointment, intrapersonal functioning, family relationships, peer relationships, school adjustment, developmental and delivery history, exposure to substances, abuse and trauma, medical and mental health history and daily functioning (9).

These interviews, although structured, can also be fluid in nature with attention being given to areas of concern. When a family brings a child in after an exposure to a motor or traffic related crash it is assumed that the child is probably having problems which led the family to seek services. Therefore during the course of the interview the clinician will want to obtain all the necessary information, but more attention will likely be spent discussing the trauma exposure along with pre and post behaviors. Understanding and knowing the criteria for various disorders, in particular PTSD, ahead of time can assist the clinician in asking certain questions related to this diagnosis to begin the process of determining if PTSD is probable.

A useful tool that a clinician can use is the structured clinical interview for the DSM-5-Clinican Version (SCID-5-CV). This tool uses a step by step process to navigate the DSM-5 criteria for certain disorders that are commonly seen (10). Included are the criteria for PTSD (10). Once a clinical interview is done a clinician can determine what assessment tools would be most appropriate for the patient and their parents to complete.

Screening assessments for PTSD

There are several PTSD screening assessments available for a clinician to use. Because the DSM-5 is fairly new, some of the PTSD tools have not been updated and are therefore still using DSM-IV criteria to assess symptoms. However, there have been studies done that have shown that there is not a significant difference in prevalence of a PTSD diagnosis whether you use the DSM-IV or DMS-5 criteria (8). Using a combination of several assessments tools may be beneficial when articulating a diagnosis. Several of these assessments are free and easily accessible to download and print off, while others must be purchased through designated assessment resources. In addition, it is important for a clinician to be aware of the age restrictions, since some of these tools are not normed for children under the age of 6 years. Some of the more popular PTSD assessments are subsequently described.

Clinician administered PTSD Scale for DSM-5-Child/Adolescent Version (CAPS-CA-5)

The CAPS-CA is considered the gold standard in assessing for PTSD in children (11). This interview tool is administered by a trained clinician and meets the PTSD criteria described in the DSM-5 for children aged of 7-18 years (12). It contains 30 items that are administered to the child or adolescent (12). The CAPS-CA-5 is comprised of standardized questions and probes that assess 20 DSM-5 PTSD symptoms (12). It also "targets the onset and duration of symptoms, subjective distress, impact of symptoms on social functioning, impairment in development, overall response validity, overall PTSD severity...and specifications for the dissociative subtype (depersonalization and derealization)" (12). In order to use this tool it requires the identification of at least one traumatic event (13). This tool can be obtained by contacting the VA's National Center for PTSD by email at ncptsd@ncptsd.org (12).

Trauma symptom checklist for children (TSCC) and young children (TSCYC)

The TSCC is designated for children from the ages 6 to 17 years and is in an interview format that measures multiple symptoms related to an exposure to traumatic event(s) (14). It is also one of the more widely used assessments that also looks at other symptoms like anger and depression (14). It has a sexual concerns component as well but this can be eliminated when screening for a specific traumatic incident like a motor or traffic related event. The TSCYC is parent or caretaker report that is used to assess PTSD symptoms in children ages 3-12 years old (15). This instrument is one of the only instruments available for preschool aged children (14). Both the TSCC and TSCYC uses the DMS-IV PTSD criteria (14, 15). This instrument can be purchased through Psychological Assessment Resources, Inc.

Traumatic events screening inventory for children - (TESI-C)

The TESI is a structured clinical interview measure for children over the age of 8 with a parent version for children under the age of 7 years (13). This tool uses DSM-IV criteria to assess for PTSD (16). The TESI-C evaluates for a variety of traumatic events that a child may encounter including accidents

(16). There is also a TESI-CRF-R version that is "more developmentally sensitive to the traumatic experiences that young children may experience" (16). This tool has a parent report version as well (TESI-PRR). The TESI-C can be obtained by contacting the VA's National Center for PTSD by email at ncptsd@ncptsd.org (16).

When bad things happen scale (WBTH)

This instrument is a self-report measure designated for children aged 8 to 13 years (17). It measures their responses to a traumatic event and uses DSM-IV criteria (13). This tool also contains a parent report version as well (17). This instrument can be obtained by contacting Kenneth E Fletcher, PhD Department of Psychiatry at Kenneth.fletcher@umassmed.edu (17).

UCLA child/adolescent PTSD reaction index for DSM-5

This instrument has recently been updated to include the DSM-5 PTSD symptom criteria. This tool includes a parent version and a self-assessment version that can be used for children ages 7-12 years and adolescents over the age of 13 years (18). The UCLA PTSD Reaction Index can "screen for the presence of any type of traumatic event" (18). It is available by contacting Preston Finley at HFinley@mednet.ucla.edu (18).

Other sources of information

In addition to a conducting a clinical interview and administering PTSD assessments, it is also suggested that additional information be obtained in order to complete a comprehensive evaluation. As stated previously, since a PTSD diagnosis requires that the symptoms being presented be a result of the experienced trauma (5), ruling in or out other factors is necessary. It is therefore suggested that a clinician have the patient participate in cognitive and academic screeners (i.e., KBIT-2, WRAT-4) to determine a person's level of functioning. Cognitive functioning can greatly impact a person's response to trauma and can play a role in understanding a patient's symptom response. It is important to note that discovering a delay in functioning or cognitive impairment does not in and of itself dismiss a PTSD diagnosis, but instead can help a clinician describe the patient's response to the trauma and it may influence how future interventions could be tailored for the patient to meet there level of ability.

It would also be beneficial if the evaluator uses affective screeners (tools that measure depression, anxiety and anger), to determine if the patient has any elevations in any of these areas. These are useful assessments because they can lead to a possible differential diagnosis or comorbid diagnosis.

In addition, a clinician may want to conduct observations (school observations), behavioral and attention and concentration screeners. All of this subsequent material can aid in developing a thorough diagnosis and subsequent treatment plan across environments. It can also rule in or out other factors that may or may not be impacting the patient.

CONCLUSION

The propensity for a child or adolescent to be exposed to a motor or traffic related crash is vast, which is also true on how they may react. Because there is such a spectrum of response when faced with a traumatic event makes diagnosing challenging. In addition a child and adolescent present with varying levels of development and environmental factors that can also be impactful. Because of these dynamics, evaluating for a mental health diagnosis is not as easy as simply looking at the symptoms and determining if a person meets the requirements of a disorder. In particular, a diagnosis of PTSD has firm criteria that is required before a patient can be formally diagnosed. An ideal way to navigate all of these elements is to conduct a comprehensive evaluation. This will provide a clinician with a detailed picture of their patient and ensure that all factors are taken into consideration. This will then aid them in articulating and developing their diagnosis and subsequent treatment plan which will likely lead to a swifter resolution of symptoms.

REFERENCES

[1] Road traffic safety. CDC Injury Center. URL: https://www.cdc.gov/safechild/Road_Traffic_Injuries/index.html.

[2] Young drivers: 2014 data. National Highway Traffic Safety Administration, National Center for Statistics and Analysis, 2016. URL: https://crashstats.nhtsa.dot.gov/Api/Public/ViewPublication/812278.

[3] Children: 2014 data. National Highway Traffic Safety Administration, National Center for Statistics and Analysis, 2016. URL: http://www-nrd.nhtsa.dot.gov/Pubs/811620.pdf%5Cnhttp://www-nrd.nhtsa.dot.gov/Pubs/809778.pdf.
[4] Romano E, Kelley-Baker T. Child passengers injured in motor vehicle crashes. J Safety Res 2015; 52:1–8.
[5] American Psychiatric Association. DSM-V. Diagnostic and statistical manual of mental disorders, 5th ed. Arlington, VA: APA, 2013.
[6] Trauma and shock. American Psychological Association. URL: http://www.apa.org/topics/trauma/
[7] Houston AA, Webb-Murphy J, Delaney E. From DSM-IV-TR to DSM-5: Changes in posttraumatic stress disorder. San Diego, CA: US Naval Center Combat Operational Stress Control (NCCOSC), 2013;1–5.
[8] Hafstad GS, Dyb G, Jensen TK, Steinberg AM, Pynoos RS. PTSD prevalence and symptom structure of DSM-5 criteria in adolescents and young adults surviving the 2011 shooting in Norway. J Affect Disord 2014;169(2014):40–6.
[9] Stephanie H. McCounaughy. Clinical interviews for children and adolescents, second ed. New York: Guilford, 2013.
[10] Structured Clinical Interview for DSM-5 (SCID-5). URL: https://www.appi.org/scid5.
[11] Hukkelberg S, Ormhaug SM, Holt T, Wentzel-Larsen T, Jensen TK. Diagnostic utility of CPSS vs. CAPS-CA for assessing posttraumatic stress symptoms in children and adolescents. J Anxiety Disord 2014;28(1):51–6. doi.org/10.1016/j.janxdis.2013.11.001.
[12] Clinician-Administered PTSD Scale for Children and Adolescents (CAPS-CA) – PTSD. National Center for PTSD, 2016 Feb 23. URL: http://www.ptsd.va.gov/professional/assessment/child/caps-ca.asp.
[13] Strand VC, Sarmiento TL, Pasquale LE. Assessment and screening tools for trauma in children and adolescents. Trauma Violence Abuse 2005;6(1):55–78.
[14] Trauma Symptom Checklist for Children (TSCC) – PTSD. National Center for PTSD, 2016 Feb 23. URL: http://www.ptsd.va.gov/professional/assessment/child/tscc.asp.
[15] Trauma Symptom Checklist for Young Children (TSCYC) – PTSD: National Center for PTSD. 2016 Feb 23. URL: http://www.ptsd.va.gov/professional/assessment/child/tscyc.asp.
[16] Traumatic Events Screening Inventory for Children (TESI-C) - PTSD: National Center for PTSD. 2016 Feb 23 [cited 2017 Jan 13]; Available from: http://www.ptsd.va.gov/professional/assessment/child/tesi.asp.
[17] When Bad Things Happen Scale (WBTH) – PTSD. National Center for PTSD, 2016 Feb 23. URL: http://www.ptsd.va.gov/professional/assessment/child/bad-things-happen.asp.
[18] UCLA Child/Adolescent PTSD Reaction Index for DSM-5 – PTSD: National Center for PTSD, 2016 Feb 23. URL: http://www.ptsd.va.gov/professional/assessment/child/ucla_child_reaction_dsm-5.asp.

In: Children and Youth
Editors: Donald E. Greydanus et al.
ISBN: 978-1-53611-102-6
© 2017 Nova Science Publishers, Inc.

Chapter 5

DIFFERENTIAL DIAGNOSIS AND COMORBID CONDITIONS

Adam J Mrdjenovich[*], PhD
Office of Research, University of Michigan,
North Campus Research Complex,
Ann Arbor, Michigan, US

There are many possible scenarios that would require a clinician to distinguish post-traumatic stress disorder (PTSD) from other mental disorders that share similar signs and symptoms. Further, psychiatric comorbidity is the rule—rather than the exception—with PTSD. This review provides information on the identification and differential diagnosis of PTSD with a focus on pediatric patients and psychological sequelae from traffic-related accidents and injuries. Age-specific features of PTSD and a PTSD subtype for preschool children are described. Factors that confound the detection and interpretation of PTSD symptoms are considered with reference to children and their parents. Common patterns of PTSD comorbidity are discussed. A summary of relevant literature is presented, from which recommendations for clinicians and future research are offered in conclusion.

---

[*] Correspondence: Adam J Mrdjenovich, PhD, University of Michigan, Office of Research, North Campus Research Complex, 2800 Plymouth Road, Building 520, Ann Arbor, MI 48109-2800, United States. Email: amrdjen@umich.edu.

INTRODUCTION

More than 700,000 children experience traumatic events of abuse or neglect each year in the United States (1). Research involving a nationally representative sample of nearly 5,000 children and adolescents aged 0-17 found that the majority (61%) of respondents had experienced or witnessed some type of victimization in the past year (2). Findings from another national study of more than 4,000 children and adolescents aged 12-17 indicate that nearly half (47%) of the participants had been exposed to violence or had experienced trauma in the form of sexual or physical assault during their lifetime (3). A plurality of these children will develop conditions such as post-traumatic stress disorder (PTSD) that can significantly impair their social, emotional, and academic functioning. Residual sequelae of childhood trauma may persist and contribute to psychological problems throughout life.

CHILDHOOD MENTAL DISORDERS: DIAGNOSTIC CHALLENGES AND DEVELOPMENTAL CONSIDERATIONS

The challenges of diagnosing mental disorders in children are widely recognized. Factors such as separation anxiety, disruptive behavior, or poor school performance can point to any number of conditions. The diagnostic process is complicated further by the potential for symptom overlap and psychiatric comorbidity. A diagnosis of PTSD, by definition, depends on a precipitating event (4). The manner in which children perceive and respond to a traumatic event is influenced largely by the nature and duration of the trauma, as well as their level of cognitive, emotional, and psychosocial development. Thus, the clinical presentation of PTSD varies considerably by developmental stage (5). This is evident in the triad of re-experiencing, avoidance, and hyper-arousal that characterizes the disorder, which does not necessarily manifest itself the same way in children as it does among adults (4, 5).

DIAGNOSTIC CRITERIA AND AGE-SPECIFIC FEATURES

The most recent revision of the *Diagnostic and statistical manual of mental disorders* (DSM-5) (4) identifies diagnostic criteria for PTSD in eight areas:

**Child Health and Human
Development Yearbook 2016**
Joav Merrick (Editor)
2017. ISBN: 978-1-53610-946-7 (Hardcover)
2017. ISBN: 978-1-53610-958-0 (e-book)

**Children and Youth:
Post-Traumatic Stress Disorder and
Motor Vehicle Crashes**
*Donald E. Greydanus, Devika Malhotra
and Joav Merrick (Editors)*
2017. ISBN: 978-1-53611-102-6 (Hardcover)
2017. ISBN: 978-1-53611-255-9 (e-book)

(A) exposure to a traumatic event; (B) re-experience such as flashbacks and nightmares; (C) avoidance of stimuli associated with the traumatic event; (D) negative alterations in cognition and mood such as dissociation, dysphoria, and emotional numbing); (E) increased arousal such as anger and hypervigilance; (F) duration of symptoms (more than one month for most); (G) significant distress or functional impairment; and (H) the disturbance cannot be attributable to the effects of a substance or another medical condition (6). Age-specific features are also described. For example, while school-aged children may not experience visual flashbacks or amnesia for aspects of a traumatic event, they do tend to experience "time skew," which refers to the mis-sequencing of trauma-related events, and "omen formation," which refers to the belief that warning signs predicted the trauma. These features are not typically observed among adults with PTSD. Additionally, school-aged children tend to exhibit posttraumatic play (i.e., a literal representation that involves compulsive repetition of some aspect of the trauma) and reenactment (i.e., a behavioral recreation of the trauma through verbalizations or drawings) (5, 7).

PTSD in preschool children

Based on research which suggested that the diagnostic criteria for PTSD needed to be more developmentally sensitive and behaviorally anchored in order to detect the disorder in younger children, DSM-5 includes a new developmental subtype called "PTSD in preschool children." Some of the general criteria for PTSD such as distress at the time of a traumatic event, an inability to recall important aspects of a traumatic event, and sensing a foreshortened future were deleted for purposes of this subtype due to developmental challenges associated with the assessment of symptoms. For other criteria, the language was modified to enhance face validity and symptom detection (e.g., "diminished interest in significant activities" may manifest among preschool children as "constricted play"; "feelings of detachment or estrangement" may manifest as "social withdrawal"; "irritability or outbursts of anger" might entail "extreme temper tantrums").

The most significant change involved the avoidance and negative cognition and mood sections, which reflect highly internalized phenomena among children. More specifically, research has shown that preschool children do not always manifest overt distress in the form of avoidance or intrusive recollections, and it is not uncommon for parents to report that they have not observed any particular affective reactions to traumatic events on the part of their child (5, 7, 8). As such, the PTSD in preschool children subtype requires only one symptom in either the avoidance or negative cognition and mood section, thus lowering the detection threshold from three symptoms in DSM-IV (8).

Prevalence and course

Although there are no definitive statistics on the prevalence of PTSD in the general population of younger children in the United States, the National Comorbidity Survey Replication Adolescent Supplement, which involves a nationally representative sample of over 10,000 adolescents aged 13-17, suggests that 5% of adolescents will meet criteria for PTSD in their lifetime (9). PTSD is more prevalent among girls than boys (8.0% vs. 2.3%) (9). Rates of PTSD are higher among children than those reported for adults (10). PTSD is a chronic disorder that, left untreated, remits at a relatively low rate (10).

Risk factors and protective factors

Factors that increase the intensity or duration of the stress response among children are associated with increased vulnerability to PTSD (7). These factors include being younger and female; having a pre-existing mental disorder; a history of previous exposure to trauma; exposure to multiple or repeated traumatic events; physical injury to the child; injury or death of a loved one; and disruption to family, home, school and/or community structure (7, 10). Conversely, increased resilience to PTSD is associated with factors such as experiencing a single traumatic event of limited duration that does *not* disrupt family, home, school, or community structure; immediate posttraumatic intervention; the ability to understand abstract concepts of trauma that would allow one to devise a rational explanation for a traumatic event; and having a nurturing family or other support system to assist the child with the immediate effects of a traumatic event and serve as a buffer against more serious sequalae (7, 10).

The detection and interpretation of PTSD symptoms

Although PTSD can be discerned readily when patients spontaneously report distressing dreams, intrusive thoughts, feelings of anger, etc., and when they present an explicit history of their exposure to traumatic events, several factors tend to confound the detection and interpretation of PTSD symptoms (11). For example, whereas the clinical presentation may consist of features associated with PTSD such as anxiety, depressed mood, and/or substance abuse, specific traumatic events might not be detected in the process of obtaining a psychiatric history. Patients might simply lack complete recollection for such events (which, incidentally, does not prevent PTSD from developing). Without a complete trauma history to aid the clinician, post-traumatic stress symptoms might be classified as part of other conditions. Even when traumatic events are acknowledged, symptoms might not appear to be connected to those events, particularly when symptoms remain latent for a period of time, or wax and wane over time. Consequently, PTSD might not be diagnosed definitively until later in the treatment process (11).

As for children, parents might not be aware that their child has been exposed to a traumatic event. Other parents might be aware of a specific event in their child's life such as a motor vehicle accident, but they may not perceive it as being particularly traumatic and/or make a connection between that event and symptoms such as avoidant behavior, tension, mood swings, tantrums, etc. on their child's part (5, 7, 12, 13). Children might lack the verbal skills to express their reactions to trauma. Children who have the requisite verbal skills may be reluctant to report such reactions because they feel frightened or ashamed. They might acknowledge that a given event would upset most children, but their responses concerning their own feelings may be more cautious (5, 7, 12, 13).

For these reasons, it is imperative that the clinician gather a careful psychiatric history, which could involve the use of standardized screening and assessment instruments. The clinician's inquiry must be age appropriate for children (e.g., tailored to ways in which fear is experienced at a given developmental stage) (5, 12). Rapport is, of course, crucial for disclosure of traumatic events that would support an accurate diagnosis of PTSD. The clinician can develop and maintain rapport with traumatized children, in part, through linguistic sensitivity and appropriate management of their own reactions to intense emotional content (e.g., avoid patronizing language and distancing gestures) (11).

DIFFERENTIAL DIAGNOSIS

There are *many* possible scenarios that would require a clinician to distinguish PTSD from other disorders that share similar signs and symptoms. Blank (11) considers the differentiation of PTSD from nearly 40 other conditions. The DSM-5 includes a comprehensive section on the differential diagnosis of PTSD with reference to psychotic, mood, anxiety, obsessive-compulsive, acute stress, adjustment, sleep, and substance-related disorders (4).

Adaptive stress response

Although PTSD can be ruled out in the true absence of trauma, a history of traumatic events does not necessarily indicate that PTSD is present. More specifically, PTSD must first be distinguished from an adaptive, appropriate, and common response to a distressing event, which would not suggest a mental disorder involving the same intensity, quantity, and diversity of symptoms as PTSD (11). Because the former is likely to subside spontaneously, psychological intervention may not be necessary (11).

General guidelines

Based on a large PTSD treatment outcome study involving military veterans, Schillaci and colleagues (14) identified relevant challenges of differential diagnosis and offered clarifying questions and guidelines for clinicians who work with PTSD populations including children. They suggest that PTSD could better account for (a) *hallucinations* attributed to a psychotic disorder, when such hallucinations constitute the re-experience of a traumatic event, (b) apparent *depressive episodes* when symptoms coalesce with a traumatic event, or when symptoms have a delayed onset but persist in the absence of depressed mood, (c) *irrational fear and avoidance* that might otherwise suggest a specific phobia, when feared objects and situations resemble—and avoidant behaviors symbolize—a specific traumatic event, and (d) *maladaptive behaviors and relational patterns* that point to a personality disorder, where trauma has occurred during critical periods of personality development (14).

Differential diagnostic considerations for children

Traumatized children are often misdiagnosed with ADHD given the attentional difficulties, distractibility, and impulsivity that come with hypervigilance (5). Because of their hyperarousal, children with PTSD as a primary diagnosis might also be (mis)diagnosed with oppositional defiant disorder or conduct disorder (10). In terms of making differential diagnoses between PTSD and conditions such as adjustment disorder, acute stress disorder, generalized anxiety disorder (GAD), and obsessive compulsive disorder (OCD) in children, Pappagallo and colleagues reiterate the implications of (a) *symptom onset and duration* (e.g., a diagnosis of adjustment disorder requires symptom onset within three months of an identifiable stressor; acute stress disorder can only be diagnosed within the first month after a traumatic event; PTSD can have a delayed onset, but symptoms must last longer than one month), (b) *the existence of a precipitating traumatic event* (GAD does not require an identifiable stressor); and (c) *intrusive thoughts* (obsessions that accompany OCD need not be related to traumatic events) (5).

COMORBID CONDITIONS

PTSD is commonly associated with psychiatric comorbidity (15-19). In a study of traumatic stress reactions to a school bus disaster, a number of children met criteria for additional diagnoses such as ADHD, oppositional defiant disorder, conduct disorder, major depressive disorder, dysthymic disorder, separation anxiety disorder, and specific phobia (15). The rate of lifetime comorbidity of any mental disorder with PTSD is approximately 80% (16). Although this figure reflects an assortment of mental disorders, research has shown that, for adults, PTSD comorbidity clusters into a small number of common patterns involving comorbid substance-related disorders, major depressive disorder, and anxiety disorders (17).

Substance-related disorders and major depressive disorder affect roughly 45% and 35%, respectively, of people with PTSD (19). Higher rates of comorbidity are generally observed among men (19). Higher comorbidity has been associated with greater severity of PTSD symptoms, increased risk of functional impairment and disability, and higher rates of suicidal ideation and parasuicidal behaviors compared to individuals with either PTSD or major depression or a substance-related disorder alone (18).

ROAD TRAFFIC ACCIDENTS, RELATED INJURIES AND PTSD

PTSD is one of the most commonly occurring mental disorders following injury (20, 21), and it is a frequent consequence of road traffic-related injury (i.e., an injury sustained in an accident as a *motor vehicle occupant*, or as a pedestrian or bicyclist *struck by a motor vehicle*) among pediatric patients (22-26). DiGallo and colleagues (22) interviewed 5-8-year-olds who had been injured in road traffic accidents and found that 14% of interviewees still suffered from moderate or severe PTSD 2-15 weeks after their accident; 17% of these children reported serious traffic-related fears. Qualitative findings indicate that some of these children were convinced they were going to die, and most of them struggled to explain what had happened during their accident (22). Parents, friends, and relatives tended to impose normality; that is, they considered the accidents to be minor, told the children their condition could have been worse, and offered relatively little opportunity for children to discuss their feelings (22).

McDermott and Cvitanovich (23) assessed the prevalence of PTSD among youth aged 8-13 years who had presented to a hospital emergency department following injury from a motor-vehicle accident and determined that 22% of participants were in the moderate or severe PTSD range, while 35% were in the mild range at three months' follow-up. Significant concordance was observed between self-reported PTSD scores on standardized assessments and clinical diagnoses of PTSD (23). In similar studies, 25% of children and adolescents aged 3-18 years (24), and 35% of children and adolescents aged 5-18 years (25), met criteria for PTSD six weeks and seven to 12 months, respectively, after they had been involved and injured in road traffic accidents. The presence of PTSD was unrelated to age, type of accident, and the nature/extent of injuries (25). However, injury severity has been a significant predictor of the number and extent of PTSD symptoms in other studies (26).

NATURE OF PTSD SYMPTOMS AMONG CHILD AND ADOLESCENT VICTIMS OF MOTOR VEHICLE ACCIDENTS

A wide range of post-traumatic symptomology was observed among a non-referred community sample of child and adolescent motor vehicle accident victims (26). The most frequently endorsed symptom was intrusive recollections of the accident triggered by cues present at the scene of the accident (34%). The most common avoidance symptom was amnesia for aspects of the accident, which some participants attributed to confusion or shock at the scene (36%). Increased irritability (18%) and sleep difficulties (16%) were the most frequently reported hyperarousal symptoms.

CONCLUSION

According to the literature, approximately 14%-35% of children and adolescents will develop PTSD secondary to road traffic accidents and related injuries (22-26). Based on a conservative annual estimate of 350,000 unintentional, nonfatal, road traffic-related injuries among youth aged 0 to 17 in the United States (27), this corresponds to as many as 122,500 individuals. Percentages are somewhat higher immediately following injury (22-26). A minority of children show considerable PTSD symptoms up to 12 months after their accident (22-26).

Clinical implications

The literature suggests that, despite the prevalence and potential severity and persistence of psychological sequela from road traffic accidents and injuries, comprehensive services are not provided for child and adolescent victims in a consistent manner (25). Thus, as part of their training, clinicians who are likely to work with children and adolescents involved in road traffic accidents should be exposed to information about victims' experiences during and immediately after an accident, as well as post-traumatic reactions that can occur even when physical injuries are relatively minor (22, 24-26). The literature recommends that physicians who treat pediatric trauma patients screen for PTSD regardless of the type of trauma and/or severity of injury (22, 24-26). Because it has such significance for subsequent coping, the psychological impact of a traffic-related accident and/or injury should be considered before patients are discharged (22, 4-26). Specialist mental health consultation should be sought regarding PTSD *as it is experienced and presented clinically by children and adolescents*. Such consultation might also entail information about related diagnoses, the challenges of differential diagnosis, and the potential for comorbid psychiatric conditions.

Implications for research

Studies have been recommended to explore the influence of developmental stage on appraisal of threat and mode of coping in response to traumatic events such as motor vehicle accidents, which could facilitate the early identification of children who may require intervention (22, 24). Similarly, it has been suggested that research should examine the long term psychological effects of road traffic accidents and injuries in an effort to identify the best ways in which children who experience chronic symptoms can be provided with effective, developmentally appropriate, interventions (25).

REFERENCES

[1] US Department of Health and Human Services Administration for Children and Families Administration on Children, Youth and Families Children's Bureau. Child maltreatment 2014. URL: http://www.acf.hhs.gov.

[2] Finkelhor D, Turner H, Ormond R, Hamby S. Violence, abuse, and crime exposure in a national sample of children and youth. *Pediatrics 2009;124(5):*1411-23.

[3] Kilpatrick D, Aciemo R, Saunders B, Resnick HS, Best CL, Schnurr PP. Risk factors for adolescent substance abuse and dependence: Data from a national sample. *J Consult Clin Psychol 2000;68(1):*19-30.

[4] American Psychiatric Association. Diagnostic and statistical manual of mental disorders, 5th edition. Washington, DC: American Psychiatric Association; 2013.

[5] Pappagallo M, Silva R, Rojas V. Differential diagnosis of PTSD in children. In: Silva R, editor. Posttraumatic stress disorders in children and adolescents. New York: WW Norton, 2004:218-36.

[6] He Q, Glas C, Veldkamp B. Assessing impact of differential symptom functioning on post- traumatic stress disorder (PTSD) diagnosis. Int J Methods Psychiatr Res 2014;23(2):131-41.

[7] Hamblen J, Barnett E. PTSD in children and adolescents. URL: http://www.ptsd.va.gov/professional/treatment/children/ptsd_in_children_and_adolescents_overview_for_professionals.asp.

[8] Meiser-Stedman R, Smith P, Glucksman E, Yule W, Dalgleish T. The posttraumatic stress disorder diagnosis in preschool and elementary school-age children exposed to motor vehicle accidents. Am J Psychiatry 2008;165(10):1326-37.

[9] Kessler R, Avenevoli S, Costello J, Georgiades K, Green JG, Gruber MJ, et al. Prevalence, persistence, and sociodemographic correlates of DSM-IV disorders in the National Comorbidity Survey Replication Adolescent Sample. Arch Gen Psychiatry 2012;69(4):372-80.

[10] Perry B. Stress, trauma, and post-traumatic stress disorder in children. URL: https://childtrauma.org/wp-content/uploads/2013/11/PTSD_Caregivers.pdf.

[11] Blank A. Clinical detection, diagnosis, and differential diagnosis of post-traumatic stress disorder. Psychiatr Clin North Am 1994;17(2):351-83.

[12] Perrin S, Smith P, Yule W. The assessment and treatment of post-traumatic stress disorder in children and adolescents. J Child Psychol Psychiatr 2000;41(3):277-89.

[13] Scheeringa M, Myers L, Putnam F, Zeanah C. Diagnosing PTSD in early childhood: An empirical assessment of four approaches. J Trauma Stress 2012;25(4):359-67.
[14] Schillaci J, Yanasak E, Adams J, Dunn N, Rehm L, Hamilton J. Guidelines for differential diagnoses in a population with posttraumatic stress disorder. Prof Psychol Res Pr 2009;40(1): 39-45.
[15] Milgram N, Toubiana YH, Klingman A, Raviv A, Goldstein I. Situational exposure and personal loss in children's acute and chronic stress reactions to a school bus disaster. J Trauma Stress 1988;1(3):339-52.
[16] Spinhoven P, Penninx B, van Hemert A, de Rooij M, Elzinga B. Comorbidity of PTSD in anxiety and depressive disorders: Prevalence and shared risk factors. Child Abuse Negl 2014; 38(8):1320-30.
[17] Galatzer- Levy I, Nickerson A, Litz B, Marmar C. Patterns of lifetime PTSD comorbidity: A latent class analysis. Depress Anxiety 2013;30(5):489-96.
[18] Hruska B, Irish L, Pacella M, Sledjeski E, Delahanty D. PTSD symptom severity and psychiatric comorbidity in recent motor vehicle accident victims: A latent class analysis. J Anxiety Disord 2014;28(7):644-9.
[19] Pietrzak R, Goldstein B, Southwick S, Grant B. Prevalence and Axis I comorbidity of full and partial posttraumatic stress disorder in the United States: Results from Wave 2 of the National Epidemiologic Survey on Alcohol and Related Conditions. J Anxiety Disord 2011;25(3):456-65.
[20] Heron-Delaney M, Kenardy J, Charlton E, Matsuoka Y. A systematic review of predictors of posttraumatic stress disorder (PTSD) for adult road traffic crash survivors. Injury 2013; 44(11):1413-22.
[21] Blanchard E, Hickling E, Taylor A, Loos W, Geradi R. Psychological morbidity associated with motor vehicle accidents. Behav Res Ther 1994;32(3):283-90.
[22] Di Gallo A, Barton J, Parry-Jones W. Road traffic accidents: Early psychological consequences in children and adolescents. Br J Psychiatry 1997;170(4):358-62.
[23] McDermott B, Cvitanovich A. Posttraumatic stress disorder and emotional problems in children following motor vehicle accidents. Aust NZ J Psychiatry 2000;34(3):446-52.
[24] De Vries A, Kassam-Adams N, Cnaan A, Sherman-Slate E, Gallagher P, Winston F. Looking beyond the physical injury: Posttraumatic stress disorder in children and parents after pediatric traffic injury. Pediatrics 1999;104(6):1293-7.
[25] Stallard P, Velleman R, Baldwin S. Prospective study of post-traumatic disorder in children involved in road traffic accidents. BMJ 1998;31/(7173):1619-23.
[26] Keppel-Benson J, Ollendick T, Benson, M. Post-traumatic stress in children following motor vehicle accidents. J Child Psychol Psychiatry 2002;43(2):203-12.
[27] Centers for Disease Control and Prevention. Leading causes of non-fatal injury reports, 2001-2014. URL: https://webappa.cdc.gov/sasweb/ncipc/nfirates2001.html.

In: Children and Youth
Editors: Donald E. Greydanus et al.

ISBN: 978-1-53611-102-6
© 2017 Nova Science Publishers, Inc.

Chapter 6

THE PSYCHOLOGICAL IMPACT OF MOTOR VEHICLE CRASHES (MVC) ON CHILDREN AND ADOLESCENTS

Roger W Apple[*], PhD

Department of Pediatric and Adolescent Medicine, Western Michigan University, Homer Stryker MD School of Medicine, Kalamazoo, Michigan, United States of America

The psychological impact of motor vehicle crashes on children and adolescents is a phenomenon that often goes under-recognized and as a result often goes untreated. There is an abundance of literature regarding the topic, however, popular culture and even medical and mental health care providers do not always seem to be paying attention. This chapter reviews the PTSD narrative section of the DSM 5 and highlights what is specifically indicated regarding children, reviews general psychological characteristics of trauma and then more specific characteristics of trauma related to motor vehicle crashes. The chapter highlights some of the most significant aspects of trauma in children including intrusive memories, rumination, thought control strategies, and the concept of social support. The overarching goal of this chapter is to increase awareness of the prevalence and significance of trauma associated with motor vehicle crashes for children and adolescents.

---

[*] Correspondence: Roger W Apple, PhD, Licensed psychologist, Assistant professor, Department of Pediatric and Adolescent Medicine, Western Michigan University, Homer Stryker MD School of Medicine, 1000 Oakland Drive, Kalamazoo, MI 49008, United States. Email: roger.apple@med.wmich.edu.

INTRODUCTION

Motor vehicle crashes have become so commonplace in United States culture that many within the culture do not consider the psychological ramifications particularly the development of posttraumatic stress disorder (PTSD). Motor vehicle crashes (MVC) can cause long term mental health problems for children and adolescents such as Acute Stress Disorder (ASD), posttraumatic stress disorder (PTSD), depressive symptoms, and numerous behavior problems that often are unrecognized and consequently receive no form of treatment or intervention (1). Many children who experience traumatic events will experience signs of distress soon after the event, usually within the first few weeks, such as avoidance behaviors, concentration and attention difficulties, withdrawal behaviors, and a loss of interest in activities (2, 3). Up to 35% of children injured in mvc have symptoms of PTSD months, or even years, after MVC (1), making it is crucial that our medical and mental health systems increase their awareness of the prevalence of PTSD related to mvc as well as improve their ability to identify traumatic symptoms in children and adolescents subsequent to MCV.

The psychological impact of motor vehicle crashes on children and adolescents is a concept that has failed to resonate with many health care and mental health care providers. It may be that motor vehicle crashes have become such a common occurrence in our daily lives that we have forgotten about the potential traumatic impact of such events. Fortunately, the general issue of trauma and children is currently receiving a significant amount of attention in the literature and in clinical practice. This review will use existing literature to help bridge the gap between general trauma literature and the literature on trauma and motor vehicle crashes involving children and adolescents in order to illuminate the psychological impact of motor vehicle crashes. Interestingly, when work began on this review it was assumed that there would be very little literature on the specific topic on traumatic stress reactions for children and adolescents related to MVC; however, that assumption was completely wrong (4-17)! While the research seems to be paying attention to this phenomenon, clinical providers and US culture as a whole does not seem to be connecting PTSD with MVC nearly as well.

Trauma can be an invisible condition debilitating the lives of countless children and adolescents who often lack the skills to communicate such complex symptoms to caregivers or healthcare providers making it essential to explicitly assess the psychological functioning of each child and adolescent that has been in a motor vehicle crash. This review will focus primarily on the psychological impact on children and adolescents resulting from motor vehicle crashes and other chapters will discuss historical background as well as specific assessment and treatment options.

GENERAL IMPACT OF TRAUMA ON CHILDREN

The impact of trauma on children and adolescents in general, or after accidental injury, has received much and growing attention in the literature (8, 18-21); however, the literature regarding the impact of trauma subsequent to motor vehicle crashes is varied often using different terminology such as road traffic accidents, road accidents, motor vehicle accidents, or motor vehicle crashes (5, 9, 10). This review will use the term motor vehicle crashes rather than motor vehicle accidents, because the term accident suggests a random act that was not intended to be harmful. This review will use current literature to draw parallels between trauma in general and trauma caused by motor vehicle crashes in order to provider a greater understanding of MVC and the traumatic impact on children and adolescents. This section will briefly review the DSM 5 narrative description of posttraumatic stress disorder, and provide a discussion regarding intrusive memories and rumination, social support, acceptance, and thought control strategies.

DSM-5 PTSD NARRATIVE DESCRIPTION

The "Diagnostic and statistical manual of mental disorders" fifth edition (DSM-5) has two criteria sets for diagnosing PTSD. one for adults, adolescents, and children over the age of six years and another for children six years and younger (22). The criteria set for children six years and younger is a helpful addition that did not previously exist in the DSM-IV-TR (23); however, this distinction is somewhat concerning considering children ages 7 years through adolescence have the same criteria as adults. For example, dissociative reactions in children may include trauma specific reenactment. Does this mean that children older than 6 years will not engage in trauma specific reenactment? It may be more appropriate to consider the child's level of developmental functioning as a guide to choosing the most appropriate criteria set; however, the distinction is an acknowledgement that there are differences in presentation of PTSD for children.

In addition to the criteria sets for PTSD, the DSM-5 also provides a narrative section immediately following the criteria sets (22). The narrative sections in the DSM-5 often help add clarity and understanding to the criteria sets and should be thoroughly reviewed. While this is also true for PTSD the narrative section for PTSD does not always clearly distinguish between children and adults. However, the following table lists information that was found in the narrative section specific to children.

Table 1. PTSD narrative section: Information specific to children

Diagnostic Features	Associated Features and Supporting Diagnosis	Prevalence
• Developmentally inappropriate sexual experiences may constitute sexually violent events without any physical violence. • Re-experiencing of the traumatic event can take the form of reenactment during play or dissociative states	• Loss of language and developmental regression	• Preschool children through adolescents have experienced lower prevalence of PTSD compared to adults; however, criteria may not have been developmentally informed.
Development and Course	**Risk and Prognostic Factors**	**Culture-Related Diagnostic Issues**
• Onset of frightening dreams that are not specific to the trauma • May express trauma through play • There may be an absence of fearful reactions • Wide range of emotional and behavioral changes • Imagined interventions during play • Limited expressive ability could lead to mood problems • Difficulty identifying the onset of symptoms • Avoidant behavior • Judge self as cowardly • Belief of social undesirability • Irritable or aggressive behavior • Reckless, thrill-seeking, or high-risk behavior	Pretraumatic • Childhood emotional problems and mental disorders • Exposure to prior trauma • Childhood adversity Peritraumatic • Witnessed threat to a caregiver Posttruamatic • Social Support / Family stability is a protective factor	• Nothing specific to children was mentioned.

Table 1. (Continued)

Gender-Related Issues	Suicide Risk	Functional Consequences of PTSD
• Prevalence is higher among females compared to males across the lifespan	• Childhood abuse can increase suicide risk. • PTSD is associated with suicide risk; however nothing specific to children was mentioned.	• Although children were not mentioned directly it was reported that functional limitation can occur in the areas of development and education.
Differential Diagnosis	**Comorbidity**	
*each of the following diagnoses should be reviewed in its entirety in the DSM-5 for information specific to children. • Adjustment disorders • Other posttraumatic disorders and conditions • Acute stress disorder • Anxiety disorders and obsessive-compulsive disorder • Major Depressive Disorder • Personality disorders • Dissociative disorders • Conversion disorder (functional neurological symptoms disorder) • Psychotic disorders • Traumatic brain injury	• Patterns of comorbidity are different from adults. • Comorbid conditions for primary include oppositional defiant disorder and separation anxiety disorder	

* Table adapted from DMS 5 section on Posttraumatic Stress Disorder.
American Psychological Assocation. Diagnostic and Statistical Manual of Mental Disorders (DSM-5®). American Psychiatric Pub; 2013. 991 p.

INTRUSIVE MEMORIES

Intrusive memories are the initial re-experiencing of trauma. Dreams, intrusive memories, and re-enactment through play as well as avoidance, numbing, psychological and physiological distress, nightmares, and flashbacks are some of the most common long-term intrusive symptoms (19, 22). In a more recent study specific to children found the main symptoms consisted of distressing and intrusive thoughts and feelings, and images through which people relive the traumatic experience (24).

Table 2. Factors influencing maintenance of intrusive memories

- Unpredictability and uncontrollability
- Perception of danger
- Causal attributions
- Effect of trauma on beliefs
- Coping strategies
- Not talking about trauma
- Safety behaviors
- Substance use/abuse
- Dissociation
- Thought suppression
- Rumination
- Guilt and Anger
- Attentional and memory biases

Table adapted from: Ehlers A, Steil R. Maintenance of intrusive memories in posttraumatic stress disorder: a cognitive approach. Behav Cogn Psychother. 1995 Jul;23(3):217–49.

Intrusive memories and rumination are commonly viewed as two of the most commonly cited predictors of posttraumatic stress disorder in children (8, 19, 24). It is extremely important to recognize that during the acute phase of a trauma intrusive memories are a normal and necessary response to trauma; however, intrusive memories that continue for a prolonged period of time can then become a maintaining factor of PTSD (19). This makes it imperative that medical and mental health care providers accurately assess for PTSD, pay attention to time frames of when the trauma occurred, and be able reassure their patients that intrusive memories are a normal reaction shortly after a trauma but also be aware that if intrusive memories are occurring months to years after a trauma they are then likely functioning in a pathological way rather than in a healing manner The following table lists possible factors which can work to maintain intrusive memories.

RUMINATION

Rumination can be thought of as a specific intrusive characteristic of PTSD and was found to be the strongest predictor of PTSD in children while reappraisal and/or reenactment was found to be associated with posttraumatic stress symptoms in both the acute phase and symptoms occurring later on (24). Such intrusive characteristics function in the onset and maintenance of PTSD in children and adolescence; however, as noted above these characteristics have a therapeutic effect early on and a possible pathological effect later on but most definitely work to maintain symptoms. "In contrast to adult findings, and at odds with our predictions, the use of reappraisal was associated with *greater* posttraumatic stress symptoms (PTSS) in the acute phase, whereas reappraisal and social support were also predictive of later PTSS" (24).

SOCIAL SUPPORT

Social support is a confusing factor when working with traumatized children and has been found to be predictive of later posttraumatic stress (24). It is unclear how social support could increase or maintain symptoms of PTSD. One idea is that children lack the cognitive skills to process information related to the trauma causing the social support to function as a reminder of the trauma (rumination) and worsen symptoms (24). Meiser-Steadmen and colleges found that a child's negative (punishment) interpretations could heighten distress thus increasing posttraumatic stress symptoms (24).

THOUGHT CONTROL STRATEGIES

Thought control strategies should be given careful consideration by medical and mental health care providers when working with children who have experienced trauma. This is because some strategies that most providers would consider helpful might actually be harmful for children. Because of this considering thought control strategies from a holistic perspective, as well as patient specific, is recommended. In fact, some studies have found no effective protective thought control strategies for children in managing intrusive thoughts during the acute phase (20, 24); however, intervention has been found effective for school age children who are at high risk for long-term psychological problems (20).

Distraction is one of the most widely used thought control strategies by children (24); however, many medical and mental health providers would consider distraction harmful or at least unhelpful. This is because of the belief that by using distraction patients consciously choose not to focus on the traumatic event making effective intervention or improvement almost impossible. However, for children reappraisal during the acute phase can actually worsen traumatic symptoms which could make distraction an acceptable thought control strategy in the short term (24); but it is still important for providers to remember that thought suppression strategies such as distraction could actually worsen symptoms in the long term.

Along with using distraction during the acute phase of a traumatic experience acceptance of intrusions and resumption of typical pre-trauma functioning may be more effective for children verses any formal thought control strategy (24). Focusing on accepting that a trauma has occurred and moving back to "normal" functioning is a strategy that can be very effective with many patients, both children and adults, because acceptance focuses on positive and healthy cognitive functioning as opposed to continuing to focus on the trauma and unhealthy cognitions. Most importantly patients may be more accepting of this approach as opposed to more traditional re-experiencing or exposure types of interventions.

Possible maladaptive thought control strategies in response to traumatic stress for children include thought suppression and distraction (depending on time of use), perseverative thinking (rumination), social control, punishment (self-blame), reappraisal, and worry (24). For children thought suppression was associated with more severe posttraumatic stress and PTSD was associated with distraction, rumination, and social withdrawal (24). In contrast to the adult population the strategy of reappraisal was associated with greater PTSS in the acute phase (24).

The general impact of trauma on children and adolescents is significant and should be taken seriously by medical and mental health care providers keeping in mind the differences noted above between how adults experience trauma and how children experience trauma. The DSM 5 provides a specific criteria set for PTSD and children which is a definite improvement from the DSM-IV-TR; however, the narrative is much more vague regarding how children experience trauma.

PSYCHOLOGICAL IMPACT OF TRAUMA FROM MOTOR VEHICLE CRASHES

One of the challenging parts of diagnosing children with PTSD is understanding the criteria in relation to motor vehicle crashes. The following table will look at the primary DSM 5 criteria for PTSD for children 6 years and younger and provide examples of what these criteria might look like when applied to motor vehicle crashes.

Table 3. Criteria for motor vehicle accidents

Criteria *Only primary criteria are presented and summarized. DSM 5 should be reviewed for detailed criteria.	Motor Vehicle Accident Example
A. Exposure to actual or threatened death, serious injury, or sexual violence.	Children's' perception of threatened death may be very different from those of adults who can understand the potential harm from a mvc better that children. Children may perceive a relatively mild mvc as a situation that threatened their life when an adult might understand their life was never in danger.
B. Presence of intrusion symptoms associated with the traumatic events.	Intrusive memories, thoughts, dreams about the specific car accident. Children may reenact the accident through play, such as crashing toy cars, which may not initially appear distressing to caregivers.
C. Persistent avoidance of stimuli or negative alterations in cognitions associated with the traumatic event.	Avoidance of riding in motor vehicles, avoidance of the location of accident, avoiding conversations, people and reminders of the mvc. Children may show increased distress when riding in motor vehicles or increased fear riding on a school bus without seatbelts.
D. Alterations in arousal and reactivity associated with the traumatic event.	After a mvc caregivers and health care provides should monitor for changes in irritable/angry outbursts, hypervigilance, exaggerated startle response, concentration problems, and sleep problems and further evaluate for the possibility of PTSD.
E. Duration is more than 1 month	Duration may be hard to assess considering that may caregivers and health care providers may not be considering PTSD subsequent to mvc's particularly since children's reactions to trauma may not always appear distressing to others.
F. Disturbance causes clinically significant distress	Distress could be apparent when riding in cars or when reminded of the accident. However, symptoms of distress could also be increased irritability, as mentioned above, which could be exacerbated by poor sleep or a decline in academic functioning. For caregivers and health care providers it is critical to monitor children for changes in behavior and to look for a clinical explanation and to not ignore mvc.
G. The disturbance is not accounted for due to the physiological effects of a substance or another medical condition.	It is always important to rule out other causes for any disturbance. It is also important to remember that not all children involved in a mvc will develop PTSD.

*Table adapted from DMS 5 section on Posttraumatic Stress Disorder.
American Psychological Assocation. Diagnostic and Statistical Manual of Mental Disorders (DSM-5®). American Psychiatric Pub; 2013. 991 p.

Characteristics of psychological impact of MVC

The psychological impact of mvc are significant and include diagnoses such as PTSD, anxiety, phobic travel anxiety, mood, adjustment disorders, and somatoform pain disorder; the DSM 5 would diagnose somatic symptom disorder with predominant pain (22, 25). In fact, PTSD is much greater from MVC (girls were found to be at higher risk than boys) than those of sport injuries and, unfortunately, the psychological need of these children often go unrecognized likely due to common frequency of MVC and a lack of awareness of the psychological consequences by health care providers (26).

For children, the development of PTSD might be different than expected. The child's perception of the incident, past experience of trauma, and appraisal of threat to life is what mediates the development of PTSD as opposed to the severity of the accident (26). Understanding this information is critical for medical and mental health care providers and makes assessing the child's perception of the incident imperative. Failure to assess children's perception of the incident can be problematic because it could lead to a diagnosis of PTSD in children that experienced a traumatic event but did not perceive it as life threatening. All too often children that have experienced anything traumatic are referred to as "trauma kids" and given a diagnosis of PTSD. This practice must stop as it not an appropriate or accurate method of assessment and it creates a bias for how children should behave if they have experienced something traumatic.

Posttraumatic stress disorder (PTSD) refers to a very specific set of symptoms and does not include other types of reactions to traumatic events such as anxiety and depression (26). Therefore, when discussing the psychological impact of MVC on children future work should likely include these factors as looking at only PTSD will not accurate describe all of the children impacted by mvc.

Negative cognitions

The concept of coping in relation to mvc may be better understood if looked at in regards to the predictors of PTSD as a psychological outcome. This allows a more holistic perspective to develop in which all of the factors influencing PTSD (positive, negative, and neutral) are considered. Cieslak discussed the influence of coping self-efficacy (CSE) on negative cognitions and the development of posttraumatic stress and found that pre trauma negative cognitions have a negative impact on the development of PTSD and indicated that "negative cognitions are the most proximal, direct predictors of posttraumatic distress, we argue that these general negative cognitions through other, trauma-specific cognitions, such as CSE" (27). Cieslak went on to report that negative cognitions that occur after a traumatic event can be measured with the Posttraumatic Cognitions Inventory (PTCI) which distinguishes between three negative cognitions: negative cognitions about self, negative cognitions about the world, and self-blame (27). On a more positive note strong self-efficacy symptoms were related to successfully managing posttraumatic stress symptoms.

Interestingly, results showed that negative cognitions at the time of mvc predicted later posttraumatic distress (27). Predictors of negative psychological outcomes following mvc include: peritraumatic response to the accident, having a diagnosable acute stress disorder, prior psychiatric difficulties, extent of physical injuries, not being responsible for the accident, and posttraumatic negative cognitions (27).

RESILIENCY IN CHILDREN AND ADOLESCENTS

All too often, within healthcare and mental health care, children who experience any challenging events are quickly diagnosed with PTSD and referred to as a *trauma kid*. Before presumptively putting these harsh labels on children it is imperative that providers become skilled and knowledgeable about how trauma impacts children, diagnostic criteria, and resiliency in order to avoid the alarming trend of over and inaccurate diagnosing of children and adolescents.

A great example of resiliency is soldiers returning home from war with only a small percentage developing the symptoms required for a diagnosis of PTSD. The same is true for children with many recovering without any intervention or psychological concerns (20). What is important here is that the majority of children are resilient and do not develop PTSD. For children, resiliency often involves a set of adaptive coping skills, as well as good mental health, which helps to prevent PTSD symptoms. It is imperative that when assessing children that medical and mental health care providers assess for resiliency and trauma symptoms to help avoid over diagnosis based on the experience of trauma alone.

SLEEP

For children problems with sleep have been found immediately, as well as year after a traumatic event, and for those diagnosed with PTSD problems with sleep is one criterion (D5) noted in the DSM-5 (22). Sleep problems are also experienced by children who have been involved in MVC. In a study by Wittman found that about 24% suffered some form of psychopathological reaction at some point six month post-accident and a 27% prevalence rate of PTSD was found one to two months after sustaining injuries in a mvc (28). Problems with prolonged subjective sleep latency were found for children diagnosed with PTSD post mvc. It was also found that sleep problems can prolong recovery and result in negative psychological outcomes as well as depression and nightmares. Acute stress disorder (ASD) and PTSD are both experienced after mvc again emphasizing the importance of expanding diagnostic efforts beyond just PTSD for children involved in mvc.

IMPACT OF CHILD AND ADOLESCENT TRAUMA ON PARENTS AND CAREGIVERS

One qualitative study analyzed teacher's narratives in relation to children who have experienced trauma and found that teachers were most concerned with being able to provide the right amount of support to children after experiencing a traumatic event (29). Considering that teachers interact with children on a daily basis they should receive sufficient training in order to help them best understand the symptoms of PTSD, how these symptoms present in an academic setting, and what might be their best response. For example, it is very common for children to not always pay attention to teachers which could result is some sort of classroom consequence or reprimand.

For children with PTSD it is very likely that the reason they were unable to pay attention was due to intrusive memories of the traumatic event. Punishing a child in this situation for not paying attention would be harmful. A good response for this child would simply be to call the child's name to get their attention and to say something like, "I just wanted to make sure you did not miss anything important." Then, at later time, or if the child appears distressed, talk to the child to see if they are ok or need any assistance such as a call home to speak with a parent to help them calm down.

CONCLUSION

The psychological impact of motor vehicle crashes on children and adolescents is often traumatic; however, does not always result in meeting all of the diagnostic criteria for posttraumatic stress disorder (PTSD). Focusing primarily on PTSD is a limitation of this chapter. Initially, the idea for this chapter was to only focus on MVC and diagnosable PTSD in order to provide a focused conversation of the phenomenon. However, by only focusing on PTSD children not meeting all of the criteria for the diagnosis might not be given full consideration by treating professionals. In order to best provide needed intervention to children who have experienced MVC is to always assess for trauma (not only PTSD) but all trauma reactions and other mental health concerns such as anxiety and depression. By taking a more holistic view of trauma will allow providers to reach more children in need of help.

REFERENCES

[1] Zehnder D, Meuli M, Landolt MA. Effectiveness of a single-session early psychological intervention for children after road traffic accidents: a randomised controlled trial. Child Adolesc Psychiatry Ment Health 2010;4:7.
[2] Kaminer D, Seedat S, Stein DJ. Postraumatic stress disorder in children. World Psychiatry 2005;4(2):121–5.
[3] Winston FK, Kassam-Adams N, Vivarelli-O'Neill C, Ford J, Newman E, Baxt C, et al. Acute stress disorder symptoms in children and their parents after pediatric traffic injury. Pediatrics 2002;109(6):e90.
[4] de Vries AP, Kassam-Adams N, Cnaan A, Sherman-Slate E, Gallagher PR, Winston FK. Looking beyond the physical injury: posttraumatic stress disorder in children and parents after pediatric traffic injury. Pediatrics 1999;104(6):1293–9.
[5] Di Gallo A, Barton J, Parry-Jones WL. Road traffic accidents: early psychological consequences in children and adolescents. Br J Psychiatry 1997;170:358–62.
[6] Di Gallo A, Parry-Jones WL. Psychological sequelae of road traffic accidents: an inadequately addressed problem. Br J Psychiatry 1996;169(4):405–7.
[7] Di Gallo A. [Injury to body and soul--psychiatric consequences of road traffic accidents in children and adolescents]. Praxis (Bern 1994) 2005;94(12):467–70.
[8] Ehlers A, Mayou RA, Bryant B. Cognitive predictors of posttraumatic stress disorder in children: results of a prospective longitudinal study. Behav Res Ther 2003;41(1):1–10.
[9] Fearnley D. Psychological consequences of road accidents in children and adolescents. Br J Psychiatry 1997;171:393-5.
[10] Keppel-Benson JM, Ollendick TH, Benson MJ. Post-traumatic stress in children following motor vehicle accidents. J Child Psychol Psychiatry 2002;43(2):203–12.

[11] Landolt MA, Vollrath M, Timm K, Gnehm HE, Sennhauser FH. Predicting posttraumatic stress symptoms in children after road traffic accidents. J Am Acad Child Adolesc Psychiatry 2005;44(12):1276–83.
[12] Mather FJ, Tate RL, Hannan TJ. Post-traumatic stress disorder in children following road traffic accidents: a comparison of those with and without mild traumatic brain injury. Brain Inj 2003;17(12):1077–87.
[13] Mehta S, Ameratunga SN. Prevalence of post-traumatic stress disorder among children and adolescents who survive road traffic crashes: a systematic review of the international literature. J Paediatr Child Health 2012;48(10):876–85.
[14] Williams JL, Rheingold AA, Knowlton AW, Saunders BE, Kilpatrick DG. Associations between motor vehicle crashes and mental health problems: data from the National Survey of Adolescents-Replication. J Trauma Stress 2015;28(1):41–8.
[15] Wittmann L, Zehnder D, Schredl M, Jenni OG, Landolt MA. Posttraumatic nightmares and psychopathology in children after road traffic accidents. J Trauma Stress 2013;23(2):232–9.
[16] Wu F, Meng W-Y, Hao C-Z, Zhu L-L, Chen D-Q, Lin L-Y, et al. Analysis of posttraumatic stress disorder in children with road traffic injury in Wenzhou, China. Traffic Inj Prev 2015 Nov 11;1–5.
[17] Zink KA, McCain GC. Post-traumatic stress disorder in children and adolescents with motor vehicle-related injuries. J Spec Pediatr Nurs 2003;8(3):99–106.
[18] Curle CE, Williams C. Post-traumatic stress reactions in children: gender differences in the incidence of trauma reactions at two years and examination of factors influencing adjustment. Br J Clin Psychol 1996;35(Pt 2):297–309.
[19] Ehlers A, Steil R. Maintenance of intrusive memories in posttraumatic stress disorder: a cognitive approach. Behav Cogn Psychother 1995;23(3):217–49.
[20] Kramer DN, Landolt MA. Early psychological intervention in accidentally injured children ages 2-16: a randomized controlled trial. Eur J Psychotraumatol 2014 Jan;5.
[21] Kramer DN, Hertli MB, Landolt MA. Evaluation of an early risk screener for PTSD in preschool children after accidental injury. Pediatrics 2013;132(4):e945-51.
[22] American Psychological Assocation. Diagnostic and statistical manual of mental disorders (DSM-5®). Arlington, VA: American Psychologic Association, 2013:991.
[23] American Psychiatric Association. Diagnostic and statistical manual of mental disorders, fourth edition, text revision. Washington, DC: American Psychiatric Association, 2000:943.
[24] Meiser-Stedman R, Shepperd A, Glucksman E, Dalgleish T, Yule W, Smith P. Thought control strategies and rumination in youth with acute stress disorder and posttraumatic stress disorder following single-event trauma. J Child Adolesc Psychopharmacol 2014; 24(1):47–51.
[25] Dalal B, Harrison G. Psychiatric consequences of road traffic accidents. Consider somatoform pain disorder. BMJ 1993;307(6914):1282.
[26] Stallard P, Velleman R, Baldwin S. Prospective study of post-traumatic stress disorder in children involved in road traffic accidents. BMJ 1998;317(7173):1619–23.

[27] Cieslak R, Benight CC, Caden Lehman V. Coping self-efficacy mediates the effects of negative cognitions on posttraumatic distress. Behav Res Ther 2008;46(7):788–98.
[28] Wittmann L, Zehnder D, Jenni OG, Landolt MA. Predictors of children's sleep onset and maintenance problems after road traffic accidents. Eur J Psychotraumatol 2012 Jan 03. doi. 10.3402/ejpt.v3i0.8402.
[29] Alisic E. Teachers' perspectives on providing support to children after trauma: A qualitative study. Sch Psychol Q 2012;27(1):51-9.

In: Children and Youth
Editors: Donald E. Greydanus et al.
ISBN: 978-1-53611-102-6
© 2017 Nova Science Publishers, Inc.

Chapter 7

ASSESSMENT, EARLY INTERVENTION AND EVIDENCE-BASED TREATMENTS FOR POSTTRAUMATIC STRESS DISORDER IN CHILDREN FOLLOWING MOTOR VEHICLE ACCIDENTS

Jennifer Kuhn[*], Phd, McKenna Corlis, MA and Amy Damashek, PhD

Division of Behavioral Health, Nemours/Alfred I duPont Hospital for Children, Wilmington, Delaware and Department of Psychology, Western Michigan University, Kalamazoo, Michigan, US

Motor vehicles accidents (MVA) are one of the leading causes of injuries for children. The consequences of a MVA include physical injuries, such as broken bones or a traumatic brain injury as well as emotional injury, such as posttraumatic stress disorder (PTSD). Between 10% and 35% of children ages 2-18 years meet criteria for PTSD following a MVA, with adolescents being at higher risk for the development of PTSD. This review will focus on assessment, early intervention, and treatment of PTSD following a MVA in children and adolescents.

---

[*] Correspondence: Jennifer Kuhn, PhD, Pediatric Psychology Fellow at Nemours/Alfred I duPont Hospital for Children, Division of Behavioral Health, 1600 Rockland Road, Wilmington, DE 19803, United States. Email: jennifer.kuhn@nemours.org.

INTRODUCTION

Unintentional injuries are the number one cause of death among children ages 0-19 years and account for 9.2 million emergency room visits yearly in the United States (US) (1). Motor vehicle accidents (MVAs) are the leading cause of unintentional injury death for children between the ages of 5 and 19 years (1). Moreover, MVAs account for 8% of the nonfatal injuries in children 0-19. Fatal and nonfatal MVA injuries are most common among adolescents (1).

The consequences of an unintentional injury can include physical injury (e.g., traumatic brain injury, broken bones) as well as emotional injury (e.g., anxiety, posttraumatic stress disorder). On average, 20% of children experience posttraumatic stress disorder (PTSD) following a severe unintentional injury (2). Approximately 10% to 35% of children develop posttraumatic stress disorder following a MVA (3). Due to the large number of MVAs each year and the traumatic nature of these events, it is important to be aware of effective screening procedures, prevention approaches, and evidence-based interventions for the treatment of PTSD following MVAs.

WHAT IS POSTTRAUMATIC STRESS DISORDER?

According to the "Diagnostic and statistical manual of mental disorders" (DSM-5), children over the age of 6 years may develop symptoms of PTSD if they are exposed to actual or threatened death, serious injury, or sexual violence (5). To meet criteria for PTSD, children must evidence symptoms from several clusters, including intrusiveness, avoidance, negative cognitions and moods, as well as arousal/reactivity. Intrusion symptoms include: recurrent distressing memories or dreams related to the traumatic event or unassociated with the trauma; flashbacks in which it feels like the traumatic events are recurring; or marked physiological reactions to internal or external triggers that are related to the event.

Avoidance symptoms include avoiding the distressing memories, thoughts, or feelings of the event or external reminders of the event. Negative cognitions or moods associated with the event may manifest as: inability to remember certain aspects of the event; exaggerated negative beliefs about oneself, others, or the world; distorted cognitions about the cause of the event; a persistent negative emotional state; diminished interest in activities; feelings of detachment from others; or inability to experience positive emotions. The last symptom cluster involves changes in arousal or reactivity, which refers to: irritable behavior and angry outbursts; reckless or self-destructive behavior; hypervigilance; exaggerated startle response; problems with concentration; or sleep disturbance.

The duration of these symptoms must be greater than one month and must cause significant distress and impairment in social or other important areas of functioning (e.g., school). For children under the age of 6, only intrusion, avoidance, and alteration in arousal and reactivity are required for a diagnosis. Also, they may show more intrusion symptoms while playing, and these symptoms may not be as obviously distressing as symptoms displayed in older children.

RISK FACTORS FOR DEVELOPING PTSD FOLLOWING INJURIES

There are multiple factors that affect a child's risk for developing PTSD following an unintentional injury. Caregivers' level of posttraumatic stress symptoms following an unintentional injury is the strongest predictor of children's PTSD symptoms (6). This finding is important because it suggests that incorporating caregivers in screening and treatment is critical. The length of hospital stay following an unintentional injury and the invasiveness of medical procedures have also been found to increase children's risk for the development of PTSD (7-9).

Child characteristics such as pre-existing internalizing behavior (e.g., anxiety) and externalizing behavior (e.g., aggression), high ratings of subjective trauma severity, high heart rate in the ED following the event, and trauma-specific thoughts, cognitions, and memories have also been shown to increase the likelihood that a child will meet criteria for PTSD following an unintentional injury (4, 10-13). In addition, children of low socioeconomic status are more likely to develop PTSD symptoms following an injury. Interestingly, evidence suggests that the mechanism of injury (motor vehicle accident versus a fall) does not have a significant effect on children's risk for developing PTSD (8, 11, 14, 15).

SCREENING FOR PTSD

Given the large number of children seen in the emergency department (ED) following an unintentional injury or MVA, it is critical that children are screened and potentially identified as at risk for developing PTSD as early as possible (1). In order for screeners to become more widely used, they must be cost-effective, short, reliable, and easy to administer (16). Currently, there are several screening methods that have been found to be efficacious in assessing for PTSD symptoms immediately following an unintentional injury.

First, the Impact of Events Scale-Revised (IES-Revised) is a free 22-item self-report screener to assess PTSD symptoms in adults that has been widely used with children (17). One study found that two thirds of children assessed using the IES-Revised following a car or sporting accident were correctly identified; however, the measure was more effective when used in combination with other measures (e.g., Revised Children's Manifest Anxiety Scale) (18). However, another study found that children may have misinterpreted some of the questions on the IES-Revised, making it a less valid measure for children (19).

The Children's Revised Impact of Events Scale (CRIES) was created based on the IES and tailored to children (20). The CRIES-8 is a free 8-item self-report measure that assesses 4 symptoms of intrusion and 4 symptoms of avoidance in children above the age of 8 (20). Perrin et al. (20) found that 75-83% of children assessed using the CRIES-8 were correctly classified as having PTSD. There is a 13-item version of the CRIES that adds 5 additional questions regarding arousal symptoms. Perrin and colleagues (20) found that the CRIES-8 performs equally to the CRIES-13, and recommended that the CRIES-8 be used as a screening tool (20).

The Child Trauma Screening Questionnaire (CTSQ) is another 8-item free screener used to assess symptoms of PTSD in children following a traumatic event (16). Five questions are asked about hyperarousal, and 5 questions are asked about re-experiencing. Children answer in a yes or no format. Kenardy and colleagues (16) found this to be more efficacious than the CRIES-8. It correctly identified 82% of children who were demonstrating distressing posttraumatic stress disorder symptoms, and it correctly screened out 74% of children who did not have any posttraumatic stress disorder symptoms (16). All of these tools are all free, short, easy, and reliable.

EARLY INTERVENTION

Due to the large number of MVAs each year and the traumatic nature of these events, it is important to examine early intervention methods for children who may be at risk for developing PTSD. There is promising literature regarding early interventions that are brief and that can be utilized shortly after a trauma to prevent the development of PTSD symptoms for children at risk following an unintentional injury.

DEBRIEFING

Debriefing is frequently used with adults following traumatic events. The purpose of debriefing, also known as critical incident stress debriefing, is to provide an opportunity for people to understand what happened to them and the traumatic event that is affecting them (21). Typically, debriefing for adults occurs within 24-72 hours in a group format. Several studies have found that this standardized approach is not effective in preventing the onset of PTSD in adults and could potentially be harmful (21). Although the literature does not support the use of debriefing in adults, debriefing has been utilized with children in both individual and group settings. The core component of debriefing includes talking about the traumatic event and peoples' responses to the event shortly after the trauma (21). In general, debriefing typically starts with a brief introduction, leads into a factual reconstruction of the traumatic event from beginning to end, then leads to children's thoughts about the traumatic event and subjective appraisals of the event. Debriefing ends with normalizing reactions and psychoeducation about future reactions and coping mechanisms (22).

Studies have examined debriefing with children in multiple contexts (e.g., group versus individual, immediately following the event versus a week later), and the results have been mixed. Stallard, and colleagues (22) recruited children ages 7-18 years who presented to the ED following a motor vehicle accident. They randomly assigned children to either a control group (neutral discussion that was not accident-related) or an intervention group (a one-session debriefing protocol) four weeks after being seen in the ED as a result of a MVA. Children in the control and intervention group had similar reductions in PTSD symptoms over time, and those who participated in the debriefing session did not make any additional gains over the control group.

This suggests that debriefing may not be effective in the reduction of PTSD symptoms, but it also may not cause any harm to children.

BRIEF AND INFORMATIONAL INTERVENTIONS

Kenardy et al. (23) aimed to evaluate a cost-effective, brief, easy-to-administer information-provision intervention in the form of a booklet. They examined 103 children (aged 7-15 years) who were admitted to the Emergency Department (ED) following an unintentional injury (29% of the sample was involved in a MVA), and participants were randomly assigned to the intervention or no intervention control group. The intervention group received an 8-page booklet designed to normalize stress reactions in children following a traumatic event. The booklet provided information on where to get help, a timeline of stress reactions, and self-help advice. Children in the intervention group had a decrease in anxiety from 1-month to 6-months post-trauma while the children in the control group showed an increase in anxiety from 1-month to 6-months. However, there was no effect of the intervention on PTSD symptoms.

In addition to examining children's reactions, they examined parents' reactions and found that the intervention group had a reduction in intrusion symptoms and overall post-traumatic distress symptoms between the initial assessment and 1-month post-trauma that was greater than the reduction in symptoms found in the control group. There was a strong association between parent and child symptoms at 1-month post-trauma, suggesting that earlier intervention with both the child and parent could be beneficial in reducing the likelihood that PTSD develops. This study suggests that this information-provision intervention may be helpful in reducing symptoms of PTSD and anxiety post-trauma for both children and their parents; however, more research is needed.

BRIEF CBT TREATMENT

Kramer et al. (24) used a randomized controlled trial (RCT) to examine a brief, two-session cognitive behavioral therapy (CBT; see page 9 for additional information) treatment as an early intervention to prevent the development of psychopathology for children injured in a motor vehicle accident or who sustained a burn injury. One hundred and eight children ages 2-16 years were recruited and randomly assigned to the treatment or to a non-treatment control group. Fifty-four children were in the intervention group, and 27 of those children were in a MVA. The treatment included reconstruction of the injury in detail (using toys or drawings), identifying and modifying dysfunctional accident related appraisals, normalizing children's stress symptoms, providing coping skills to help with stress reactions, and provision of a leaflet with information about posttraumatic stress. Parents were present during the intervention.

There were no reductions in symptoms for preschool aged children. However, 7-16 year-olds in the treatment group reported less intrusion and internalizing symptoms (e.g., anxiety) at the 3-month follow-up. This is the first study examining this brief, two-session treatment, and while it shows promising results, more research is needed to see if the findings can be replicated.

COMPUTERIZED TREATMENT

Cox et al. (25) recruited 56 children ages 7-16 in an ED setting who sustained an unintentional injury (e.g., MVA, fall, burn). This study utilized an intervention that included the booklet from the Kenardy and colleagues (discussed above, 23) study along with a web-based intervention (http://kidsaccident.psy.uq.edu.au). Children and their parents were randomly assigned to a treatment (29 participants) or an assessment only control group (27 participants), and the treatment group was provided with these materials to use at home. The parent component included a booklet that contained information on normative reactions to trauma, a timeline of reactions, ways to assist their child in their recovery, and a section for the parents to encourage positive coping mechanisms for themselves and their children.

The children's website included information designed to normalize and promote recovery and included brief explanations and examples of coping mechanisms, incorporating pleasant events into daily life, reflecting on the event, problem solving, and finding help. Results of this study found a significant decrease in children's anxiety and a mild reduction in depression, anger, and posttraumatic stress symptoms for children who were in the treatment group. This intervention is brief and easy for families to use in the comfort of their own home and shows promise as an early intervention to help prevent the development of PTSD or other psychopathology following trauma.

CONCLUSIONS ON EARLY INTERVENTION

Early intervention in children following exposure to a motor vehicle accident may significantly decrease their likelihood of developing PTSD or another related mental health outcome (e.g., anxiety, depression). Debriefing has not shown promising results, but brief interventions in the form of booklets and websites as well as a brief CBT treatment has shown promising findings. The common link between these treatments is that parents were involved in the treatment, and that much of the treatment focused on normalizing reactions and providing coping mechanisms for children and their parents. It will be important to consider using these brief, early interventions with children who are at risk for developing PTSD following a motor vehicle accident in an attempt to prevent the development of PTSD or other psychopathology.

EVIDENCE-BASED TREATMENTS FOR PTSD IN CHILDREN

While early interventions have shown promise, some children who meet criteria for PTSD or whose symptoms are more severe may require more intensive treatment following a traumatic event. However, few known evidence-based treatment options are available for children with symptoms of PTSD following a traumatic event (26). The strongest evidence is based on the cognitive model of posttraumatic stress disorder (11), which posits that cognitive distortions associated with the trauma lead to persistence of symptoms.

Cognitive behavioral therapy (CBT) and more specifically, trauma-focused cognitive behavioral therapy (TF-CBT), has demonstrated efficacy across trauma types and populations. TF-CBT, developed by Cohen and colleagues (27), was initially intended to decrease PTSD symptoms after experiencing child maltreatment by helping children learn to regulate their emotions and learn coping strategies (28). Subsequent research supports the efficacy of TF-CBT across a range of trauma types (e.g., physical, sexual, natural disaster, accidents) and populations (e.g., young children and adolescents) (28).

While some interventions vary in the exact components included in the treatment, most include psychoeducation about trauma and its consequences, incorporation of parents and children in treatment, and exposure to traumatic memories (26).

CBT

The effectiveness of CBT as an appropriate treatment for children with PTSD has been studied in multiple formats. For example, a case study with two child participants demonstrated a reduction in PTSD symptoms following participation in CBT (29). One participant's symptoms followed a MVA specifically. Both participants engaged in 12 sessions of a manualized treatment: the first six sessions provided awareness training to recognize and judge symptoms and taught relaxation strategies to manage symptoms. The next four sessions required in- and out- of session exposures to memories of the trauma. The last two sessions discussed relapse-prevention strategies, reviewed the session materials, and celebrated with a graduation.

Other researchers have also found support for CBT following exposure to a single-incident trauma (e.g., motor vehicle accident, interpersonal violence, or witnessing violence) (30). They recruited 24 participants ages 8 to 18 from a trauma clinic. Prior to treatment intervention, they monitored participants' symptoms for four weeks. Following this period, almost a quarter of the participants no longer met criteria for PTSD. The remaining participants who still met criteria for PTSD then participated in CBT or a wait-list control group. CBT followed a similar structure to that which was described above and included: psychoeducation, exposure, re-engagement in activities, cognitive restructuring, and stimulus discrimination (regarding reminders of the trauma). Following the 10-week protocol, participants in the CBT group showed greater reductions in PTSD symptoms, depression, and anxiety, with an increase in functioning compared to the control group. These effects were observed at the end of treatment and maintained at the 6-month follow-up.

Of particular interest, they also found that participants' cognitive misappraisals of the trauma partially mediated the effect of therapy on PTSD symptoms. This highlights a critical variable to consider when designing and implementing therapies for children with PTSD. Approximately half of the participants' traumas were MVAs, but results were not examined differentially by treatment group. Additionally, given the age of youth with whom they worked, results may not generalize to younger children.

TF-CBT

Trauma-focused cognitive behavioral therapy (TF-CBT) is a specific CBT therapy that has been researched extensively and is well supported for treating child trauma symptoms. The intervention was developed for children who have experienced child abuse, but has been successfully used for other types of trauma as well. The acronym CRAFTS captures the key values of TF-CBT: components based, respectful of cultural values, adaptable and flexible, family focused, therapeutic relationship is central, and self-efficacy is emphasized (27).

The therapy includes three overarching phases including stabilization, creation of a trauma narrative, and integration/consolidation (31). Within those stages are eight specific components that are addressed including: psychoeducation, parenting skills, relaxation skills, affect modulation, cognitive processing, trauma narrative, in-vivo mastery, conjoint child-parent sessions, and enhancing future safety and development. A brief review of the different stages of treatment is provided below (for a full description, see references 27 and 31).

Stabilization, which may take anywhere from 4-12 sessions, addresses the first five components (31). Although psychoeducation is the first component addressed in TF-CBT, it remains a recurrent theme throughout treatment. As described by Cohen and colleagues (27), the goal of psychoeducation is to inform families about common traumas and trauma responses. Normalizing responses to trauma and validating patients' experiences is important to establishing rapport and giving families hope. Psychoeducation can also facilitate recognition of triggers related to the patient's individual experience, and recognizing appropriate versus maladaptive cognitions surrounding the trauma.

Because PTSD often includes symptoms of hypervigilance and anxiety, teaching patients relaxation strategies is imperative. Suggested relaxation techniques include deep breathing, progressive muscle relaxation, and mindfulness. To manage affective symptoms, treatment also increases awareness of symptoms, encourages the use of positive self-talk, and builds problem-solving and social skills (27). Finally, youth with PTSD often have maladaptive cognitions surrounding the trauma. Therefore, identifying and challenging those inaccurate cognitions is an important part of treatment (27).

The trauma narrative phase requires patients to gradually narrate and process their traumas (31). This is a gradual exposure to memories of the trauma to help process the event, as well as the associated thoughts and feelings. Exposure usually occurs in multiple formats, with the child writing about the trauma first and gradually expanding on it to include more detail. The child also discusses the trauma with the therapist and often the primary caregiver in increasing detail over the course of four to six sessions.

Cohen et al. (27) describe the final stage, integration/consolidation which lasts four to six sessions, as addressing the final three components. They explain in-vivo mastery as a gradual process designed to extinguish the fear and avoidance of trauma memories and triggers. Importantly, therapists must appropriately help patients identify real versus perceived threats. Fear of stimuli presenting real danger is adaptive; however, patients with PTSD often associate non-threatening stimuli with the trauma. This type of fear and subsequent avoidance is considered maladaptive and should be addressed in therapy (27).

The parenting portion of the therapy focuses on providing education and training in responding to children's dysregulation and behavior problems in a trauma-informed way (31). The conjoint child-parent sessions occur in phase three; individual session time is divided equally between parents and children until that point. During the conjoint sessions, the child shares their trauma narrative with the parent(s). Conjoint sessions can facilitate communication and improve parents' understanding of their children's experiences. Finally, enhancing future safety and development is an important piece of TF-CBT (31). Patients learn skills to minimize the risk of experiencing another trauma. Families also discuss relapse prevention strategies to maintain functioning.

To our knowledge, there have not been RCTs examining the efficacy of TF-CBT in participants who only experienced a motor vehicle accident. However, there are numerous studies supporting the efficacy of TF-CBT using participants who experienced other traumatic events (32, 33). In a review of interventions for children and adolescents with PTSD, Morina and colleagues (33) found that TF-CBT was the most frequently researched compared to other treatments, and consistently showed medium to large effect sizes against wait-list and active control groups.

In addition, a meta-analysis examining ten studies using TF-CBT found moderate pooled effect sizes for TF-CBT's efficacy in the reduction of PTSD symptoms against comparison groups immediately following treatment, with slight decreases in effect sizes at 12-month follow-up (32). Importantly, the effectiveness of TF-CBT has been demonstrated across a variety of ages, including young children (34) and adolescents (35). Additionally, TF-CBT has demonstrated efficacy across different formats and settings, such as a stepped-care format, in groups, and in schools.

Stepped-care TF-CBT

Given data suggesting that many PTSD symptoms may naturally decrease in the weeks following a trauma (30), a stepped-care approach may be an efficient, cost-effective method of alleviating trauma symptoms. A stepped-care approach organizes stages of treatment hierarchically. If symptoms remit quickly, patients phase out at an earlier stage; if symptoms persist, patients progress to a more intensive phase (36).

Salloum et al. (37) conducted an RCT comparing a stepped-care TF-CBT (SC-TF-CBT) versus TF-CBT for participants experiencing post-traumatic stress symptoms. The first step of the SC-TF-CBT required three therapist sessions and 11 parent-child sessions in the home. Throughout these sessions, participants received psychoeducation, learned relaxation strategies, and also watched videos modeling imaginal and in vivo exposures. If children were responsive to this step, families participated in a 6-week maintenance stage. If children did not respond after the first step, they progressed to step two and participated in nine TF-CBT sessions.

Results from this study indicated few differences on outcome measures between the two groups, and SC-TF-CBT was much more cost-effective. Importantly, a majority of children in the SC-TF-CBT group responded to treatment after step one. While these results suggest a stepped-care approach may be an efficient and cost-effective method for alleviating symptoms related to trauma, future research should replicate these findings with larger and more diverse samples.

Group-based TF-CBT

There is also evidence that TF-CBT is effective when delivered in a group setting. The TF-CBT group therapy protocol is implemented similarly to individual services. Treatment usually runs 10-14 sessions and groups are balanced by age and gender. Importantly, research supports that both mixed- and same-sex groups are equally effective (38). While it appears that TF-CBT may be effective regardless of treatment mode, future research should conduct randomized controlled trials comparing TF-CBT conducted in an individual versus group format. As highlighted by Deblinger and colleagues (38), group treatment can have a multitude of benefits including facilitating enrollment in services and decreasing wait-time for service involvement. Additionally, group therapy is often a very cost-effective method for therapy delivery.

School based interventions

Cognitive Behavioral Intervention for Trauma in Schools (CBITS) is an evidence-based treatment used to treat children in their own school who display symptoms of PTSD after exposure to violence (39). CBITS was originally created for 4th to 8th grade children, but it has been adapted for Kindergarten through 5th grade children as well. CBITS consists of 10 one-hour group sessions, 1-3 individual sessions for children to discuss their trauma, 2 group educational sessions for parents, and 1 group educational session for teachers. Four to six children per group is the ideal size, and school-based mental health professionals are the clinicians for the group.

The goals of CBITS are to provide early intervention to children in a setting that is familiar, to reduce psychological reactions to a trauma (e.g., PTSD symptoms, anxiety, depression), and promote resilience factors to promote better functioning in school, home, and with peers. CBITS uses a cognitive-behavioral approach to treatment and incorporates many of the same components as TF-CBT including psychoeducation about trauma, relaxation training, identifying and challenging dysfunctional thinking, approaching rather than avoiding trauma, assessing safety of situations, and developing a trauma narrative (39).

CBITS has been shown to be an effective method for early intervention in children with PTSD in a setting that is familiar and easy to access (i.e., their school). Stein et al. (40) randomly assigned participants to an early intervention CBITS group or a delayed intervention CBITS group. At 3-month follow up, the early intervention group showed a 64% reduction in PTSD symptoms versus a 34% reduction in the delayed intervention group. In addition, those in the early intervention group reported a significant reduction in depression and psychosocial dysfunction. At 6-month follow up, the early intervention group maintained their decreased symptoms, and the delayed intervention group displayed a significant reduction in symptoms over time.

CBITS has also been compared to school-based TF-CBT (41). Students who survived Hurricane Katrina were randomized to either individual TF-CBT with parent involvement or CBITS. Students who participated in CBITS attended 10-group sessions and 1-3 individual sessions. Students in CBITS saw improvements in PTSD and depression scores, while those in TF-CBT only saw improvements in PTSD symptoms. Additionally, the authors concluded CBITS was a better option for families who did not have the desire or resources to participate in the more traditional form of therapy. Based on these findings, it appears that school-based interventions, specifically CBITS, may be an effective way to treat trauma symptoms.

Other treatments

Eye Movement Desensitization and Reprocessing (EMDR) is a commonly used, evidence-based treatment for PTSD in adults, and it has shown promising results for children with PTSD (43). Treatment includes 8 phases, and the critical part of the intervention is bilateral stimulation of the brain using visual, auditory, and tactile stimuli while discussing the traumatic event (26). A combination of desensitization and exposures are utilized throughout the treatment. For example, children who participate in this treatment may complete eye movements while recalling the traumatic event and their thoughts, feelings, and body sensations (43).

One RCT specifically examined a 4-session EMDR treatment for 27 children ages 6-12 who had PTSD symptoms following a motor vehicle accident (43). Children were assigned to a treatment condition or a wait-list control condition. Results showed that while reductions in PTSD symptoms were not statistically significant from pre-intervention to post-intervention, there was a decrease in PTSD symptoms in just 4 sessions that was greater than the control group. These improvements in PTSD symptoms maintained at a 3-month follow-up. This brief, exposure-based treatment shows promise in reducing PTSD symptoms in children following MVAs. However, more research examining the effects of EMDR for children with PTSD symptoms following MVAs is needed.

CONCLUSION

Motor vehicle accidents account for 8% of the nonfatal injuries in children 0-19 and account for the greatest number of nonfatal injuries among adolescents ages 15-19 years (1). Between 10% to 35% of children develop posttraumatic stress disorder as a result of MVAs (3), indicating that early screening and intervention to prevent the development of symptoms is critical in reducing the rates of PTSD in children following MVAs. If a child is seen in an ED or primary care visit following a MVA, it will be beneficial for providers or staff to implement a brief screener (e.g., CRIES-8, CTSQ) to determine which children may be at a high risk for the development of psychopathology following a trauma. Early screening may lead to more appropriate referrals so that children can receive treatment as quickly as possible. Researchers have found promising results with web-based and brief CBT interventions provided shortly after an injury occurrence (23-26).

With regard to children who do develop PTSD as the result of a MVA, CBT interventions have strong empirical support in terms of reducing PTSD symptoms (26). There is a range of research supporting the efficacy and generalizability of CBT for children with PTSD; however, it has not been rigorously tested specifically for children who experienced a MVA. One study did examine the efficacy of EMDR with children who experienced a MVA; the authors found a reduction in symptoms, but it was not statistically significant (43).

Although CBT interventions have not been tested specifically with children who experienced MVAs, it is likely that these treatments will be effective if used with children who have been in a MVA. Indeed, CBT has been found to be effective for children who experienced a wide range of traumas (30). However, it is possible that there may be aspects of MVAs that are unique that need to be addressed in therapy, such as a resulting injury or disability.

Future directions for PTSD treatment in children following MVAs should focus on increasing screening for PTSD in the ED setting or in primary care offices in order to detect children who are at risk as early as possible. Another future direction may be to incorporate elements of CBT (e.g., psychoeducation, relaxation training) in shorter, briefer formats in primary care settings to make such resources more accessible. This will be helpful in reaching a large number of children who are experiencing symptoms of PTSD following a MVA (44). By implementing evidence-based interventions in a setting that could reach significantly more children, rates of PTSD could be reduced significantly for children following MVAs.

REFERENCES

[1] Borse NN, Gilchrist J, Dellinger AM, Rudd RA, Ballesteros MF, Sleet DA. Unintentional childhood injuries in the United States: Key findings from the CDC childhood injury report. J Safety Res 2009;40(1):71–4.

[2] Ostrowski SA, Ciesla JA, Lee TJ, Irish L, Christopher NC, Delahanty DL. The impact of caregiver distress on the longitudinal development of child acute post-traumatic stress disorder symptoms in pediatric injury victims. J Pediatr Psychol 2011;36(7):806–15.

[3] Landolt M, Vollrath M, Timm K, Gnehm H, Sennhauser F. Predicting posttraumatic stress symptoms in children after road traffic accidents. J Am Acad Child Adolesc Psychiatry 2005;44(12):1276–83.

[4] Meiser-Stedman R, Glucksman E, Yule W, Dalgleish T. The posttraumatic stress disorder diagnosis in preschool- and elementary school-aged children exposed to motor vehicle accidents. Am J Psychiatry 2008;165(10):1326–37.

[5] American Psychiatric Association. Diagnostic and statistical manual of mental disorders, 5th edition. Washington, DC: American Psychiatric Association, 2013.

[6] Bronner MB, Knoester H, Bos AP, Last BF, Grootenhuis MA. Posttraumatic stress disorder (PTSD) in children after paediatric intensive care treatment compared to children who survived a major fire disaster. Child Adolesc Psychiatry Ment Health 2008;2(1):9.1.

[7] Bryant B, Mayou R, Wiggs L, Ehlers A, Stores G. Psychological consequences of road traffic accidents for children and their mothers. Psychol Med 2004;34(2):335–46.

[8] Keppel-Benson JM, Ollendick TH, Benson MJ. Post-traumatic stress in children following motor vehicle accidents. J Child Psychol Psychiatry Allied Discip 2002;43(2):203–12.

[9] Olsson KA, Kenardy JA, De Young AC, Spence SH. Predicting children's post-traumatic stress symptoms following hospitalization for accidental injury: Combining the Child Trauma Screening Questionnaire and heart rate. J Anxiety Disord 2008;22(8):1447–53.

[10] Cox CM, Kenardy JA, Hendrikz JK. A meta-analysis of risk factors that predict psychopathology following accidental trauma. J Spec Pediatr Nurs 2008;13(2):98–110.

[11] Ehlers A, Clark DM. A cognitive model of posttraumatic stress disorder. Behav Res Ther 2000;38(4):319–45.

[12] Scheeringa MS, Wright MJ, Hunt JP, Zeanah CH. Factors affecting the diagnosis and prediction of PTSD symptomatology in children and adolescents. Am J Psychiatry 2006;163(4):644–51.

[13] Winston FK, Kassam-Adams N, Garcia-Espana F, Ittenbach R, Cnaan A. Screening for risk of persistent posttraumatic stress in injured children and their parents. JAMA 2003;290(5):643–9.

[14] Nugent NR, Ostrowski S, Christopher NC, Delahanty DL. Parental posttraumatic stress symptoms as a moderator of child's acute biological response and subsequent posttraumatic stress symptoms in pediatric injury patients. J Pediatr Psychol 2007;32(3):309–18.

[15] Zink KA, McCain GC. Post-traumatic stress disorder in children and adolescents with motor vehicle-related injuries. J Spec Pediatr Nurs 2003;8(3):99–106.

[16] Kenardy J, Spence SH, Macleod AC. Screening for posttraumatic stress disorder in children after accidental injury. Pediatrics 2006;118(3):1002–9.

[17] Weiss DS, Marmar CR. The impact of event scale-revised in assessing psychological trauma and PTSD: A practitioner's handbook. New York: Guilford, 1997.

[18] Stallard P, Velleman R, Salter E, Howse I, Yule W, Taylor G. A randomised controlled trial to determine the effectiveness of an early psychological intervention with children involved in road traffic accidents. J Child Psychol Psychiatry Allied Discip 2006;47(2):127–34.

[19] Yule W, Udwin O. Screening child survivors for post-traumatic stress disorders: experiences from the "Jupiter" sinking. Br J Clin Psychol 1991;30(Pt 2):131–8.

[20] Perrin S, Meiser-Stedman R, Smith P. The Children's Revised Impact of Event Scale (CRIES): Validity as a screening instrument for PTSD. Behav Cogn Psychother 2005;33(4):487.
[21] Stallard P, Salter E. Psychological debriefing with children and young people following traumatic events. Clin Child Psychol Psychiatry 2003;8(4):445–57.
[22] Stallard P, Velleman R, Salter E, Howse I, Yule W, Taylor G. A randomised controlled trial to determine the effectiveness of an early psychological intervention with children involved in road traffic accidents. J Child Psychol Psychiatry Allied Discip 2006;47(2):127–34.
[23] Kenardy J, Thompson K, Le Brocque R, Olsson K. Information-provision intervention for children and their parents following pediatric accidental injury. Eur Child Adolesc Psychiatry 2008;17(5):316–25.
[24] Kramer DN, Landolt MA. Early psychological intervention in accidentally-injured children ages 2-16 years: a randomized controlled trial. Eur J Psychotraumatol 2014;5:24402.
[25] Cox CM, Sci B, Kenardy JA, Hendrikz JK. A randomized controlled trial of a web-based early intervention for children and their parents following unintentional injury. J Pediatr Psychol 2010;35(6):581–92.
[26] Landolt MA, Kenardy JA. Evidence based treatments for trauma-related psychological disorders: A practical guide for clinicians. New York: Springer, 2015:523.
[27] Cohen JA, Mannarino AP, Deblinger E. Treating trauma and traumatic grief in children and adolescents: A clinician's guide. New York: Guilford, 2006.
[28] Ramirez de Arellano M, Lyman DR, Jobe-Shields L, George P, Dougherty RH, Daniels AS, et al. Trauma-focused cognitive-behavioral therapy for children and adolescents: Assessing the evidence. Psychiatr Serv 2014;65(5):591–602.
[29] Scheeringa MS, Salloum A, Arnberger RA, F.Weems C, Amaya-Jackson L, Cohen JA. Feasibility and effectiveness of cognitive–behavioral therapy for posttraumatic stress disorder in preschool children: Two cases. J Trauma Stress 2007;20(4):631–6.
[30] Smith P, Yule W, Perrin S, Tranah T, Dalgleish T, Clark DM. Cognitive-behavioral therapy for PTSD in children and adolescents. J Am Acad Child Adolesc Psychiatry 2007;46(8):1051–61.
[31] Cohen JA, Mannarino AP. Trauma-focused cognitive behavior therapy for traumatized children and families. Child Adolesc Psychiatr Clin North Am 2015;24:557-70.
[32] Carly CE, McMillen JC. The data behind the dissemination: A systematic review of trauma-focused cognitive behavioral therapy for use with children and youth. Child Youth Serv Rev 2012;34(4):748–57.
[33] Morina N, Koerssen R, Pollet TV. Interventions for children and adolescents with posttraumatic stress disorder: A meta-analysis of comparative outcome studies. Clin Psychol Rev 2016;47:41–54.
[34] Scheeringa MS, Weems CF, Cohen JA, Amaya-Jackson L, Guthrie D. Trauma-focused cognitive-behavioral therapy for posttraumatic stress disorder in three-through six year-old children: A randomized clinical trial. J Child Psychol Psychiatry 2011;52(8):852–60.
[35] Jensen TK, Holt T, Ormhaug SM, Egeland K, Granly K, Hoaas LC, et al. A randomized effectiveness study comparing trauma-focused cognitive behavioral therapy with therapy as usual for youth. J Clin Child Adolesc Psychol 2014;43(3):356–69.

[36] O'Donohue WT, Draper C. Stepped care and e-health: Practical applications to behavioral disorders. New York: Springer, 2011.
[37] Salloum A, Wang W, Robst J, Murphy TK, Scheeringa MS, Cohen JA, et al. Stepped care versus standard trauma-focused cognitive behavioral therapy for young children. J Child Psychol Psychiatry 2015;57(5);614-22.
[38] Deblinger E, Pollio E, Dorsey S. Applying trauma-focused cognitive-behavioral therapy in group format. Child Maltreat 2016;21(1):59–7.
[39] Jaycox LH, Langley AK, Stein BD, Kataoka-Endo SH, Wong M. Early intervention for abused children in the school setting. In: Reece RM, Hanson RF, Sargent J, eds. Treatment of child abuse: Common ground for mental health, medical, and legal practitioners. Baltimore, MD: Johns Hopkins University Press, 2014:76–85.
[40] Stein BD, Jaycox LH, Kataoka SH, Wong M, Tu W, Elliott MN, et al. A mental health intervention for schoolchildren exposed to violence: a randomized controlled trial. JAMA 2003;290(5):603–11.
[41] Jaycox LH, Cohen JA, Mannarino AP, Walker DW, Langley AK, Gegenheimer KL, et al. Children's mental health care following Hurricane Katrina: A field trial of trauma-focused psychotherapies. J Trauma Stress 2010;23(2):223–31.
[42] Ruggiero KJ, Morris TL, Scotti JR. Treatment for children with posttraumatic stress disorder: Current status and future directions. Clin Psychol Pract 2001;8(2):210–27.
[43] Kemp M, Drummond P, McDermott B. A wait-list controlled pilot study of eye movement desensitization and reprocessing (EMDR) for children with post-traumatic stress disorder (PTSD) symptoms from motor vehicle accidents. Clin Child Psychol Psychiatry 2010;15:5–25.
[44] Sabin JA. Primary care utilization and detection of emotional distress after adolescent traumatic injury: identifying an unmet need. Pediatrics 2006;117(1):130–8.

In: Children and Youth
Editors: Donald E. Greydanus et al.
ISBN: 978-1-53611-102-6
© 2017 Nova Science Publishers, Inc.

Chapter 8

YOUTH MOTOR-VEHICLE COLLISION SURVIVORS IN THE CLASSROOM

A Benton Darling[*], MA
Department of Counseling, Rehabilitation Counseling,
and Counseling Psychology, College of Education
and Human Services, West Virginia University, Morgantown,
West Virginia, US

Many children and adolescents experience psychological consequences resulting from traumatic events that can impair their development in key areas of functioning. Involvement in a motor vehicle collision (MVC) may compromise children's maturation in social, emotional, behavioral, and academic domains. Approximately one-third of youth MVC survivors experience Posttraumatic Stress Disorder symptomatology. This review serves educators by providing an overview of trauma-related disorders among school-age children. As teachers are the primary caregivers in classrooms, it is useful to understand how trauma impacts children's abilities to learn, perform, and interact in academic environments. This review aims to describe signs and symptoms of trauma- and stressor-related disorders to assist educators in identifying and responding to at-risk children. The unique needs of youth MVC survivors are discussed to aid educators in conceptualizing classroom

---

[*] Correspondence: A Benton Darling, MA, West Virginia University, College of Education and Human Services, Department of Counseling, Rehabilitation Counseling, and Counseling Psychology, 502 Allen Hall, PO Box 6122, Morgantown, WV 26505-6122, United States. Email: bendarling15@gmail.com.

behavior and to equip them with knowledge to inform their interventions. Next, the author describes how parental involvement can be managed effectively during the recovery process. Finally, a model for trauma-sensitive classrooms is presented, as well as implications for teachers who support and educate youth survivors of trauma.

INTRODUCTION

Motor vehicle collisions (MVCs) are the leading cause of unintentional fatal injury among children and adolescents in the United States. In 2014, 2,694 children under the age of 18 years were killed in MVCs (1). MVCs also represent the leading cause of death for older adolescents and young adults between the ages of 16 and 24 years. In the three-year period from 2012 to 2014, approximately 3,230 deaths occurred each year on average, representing nearly 25% of all fatalities for this age group (2). While MVC fatality rates among children are strikingly high, many more children and adolescents suffer nonfatal motor-vehicle-related injuries. In the United States in 2014, approximately 750,000 children younger than 19 were injured in transportation-related collisions (3). This includes youth occupants of motor vehicles as well as children injured in traffic crashes as pedestrians and bicyclists.

Grade school children spend about 30% of each day at school during the academic year, which spans roughly half of every year for many children between the ages of 5 and 18 years (4). An abundance of growth and development occurs in numerous domains during these formative years (i.e., physical, social, emotional, behavioral), all of which may be negatively affected by the occurrence of a MVC. Schools also represent the central community for many children whereby they interact daily with peers and caring adults. For the many children who unfortunately are injured in MVCs each year, their injury and recovery may compromise maturation in key areas of functioning. For example, considerable absences may accrue concurrent with lengthy hospital stays, causing children to fall behind their peers in academic learning. For children who are able to return to school relatively quickly, the physical and psychological consequences that they endure may be longstanding and inhibit their ability to succeed in educational settings.

In the event that youth MVC survivors enter their classrooms, it behooves educators to understand the unique needs of these students. Teachers are the primary caregivers in these settings and they are encouraged to consider how

MVC-related trauma affects children's abilities to learn and function in school. This knowledge may frame the interaction between teachers and students as to how teachers respond to often challenging and confusing behaviors (5). It may also aid in determining necessary and appropriate accommodations, as well as inform educators' collaboration with caregivers and mental health professionals. A trauma sensitive school environment may be the difference between trauma survivors reaching their maximum academic potential or falling through the cracks.

TRAUMA- AND STRESSOR-RELATED DISORDERS

Posttraumatic stress disorder (PTSD) is characterized by three symptom clusters that may be perceptible to educators in academic settings: 1) re-experiences or intrusions, 2) hyperarousal, and 3) avoidance. A diagnosis of PTSD requires exposure to actual or threatened death or serious injury that causes significant distress or impairment in key areas of functioning. Symptoms must persist for a minimum of one month following exposure to a traumatic event (6). A motor vehicle collision is precisely the type of traumatic event from which PTSD symptomatology may develop.

Research has shown that in a sample of children involved in traffic collisions, re-experience was the most commonly reported PTSD symptom, endorsed at a rate greater than 50% (8). Within the re-experience symptom cluster are intrusive recollections, which were reported to occur most frequently, followed first by upsetting reminders of the collision and then by discomforting flashbacks. The second most frequently endorsed PTSD symptom was hyperarousal, which includes increased irritability and temper tantrums, sleep problems, hyper-alertness, and decreased concentration. Lastly, avoidance symptoms were reported, including amnesia (i.e., forgetfulness) for parts of the collision and the avoidance of collision-related situations (8).

In a review of 12 studies that assessed the psychological consequences of MVCs among children and adolescents, PTSD was identified in 27% of collision survivors (9). Individual studies of PTSD prevalence however, have reported rates as high as 35% in children six weeks after the collision, with symptoms considered by these children to be sufficient to interfere with daily functioning in the classroom (10). Gender appears to be an important determinant of PTSD onset; Females are three times more likely than males to develop PTSD (9). It is therefore prudent for teachers to be aware of this and similar risk factors, which are discussed in detail later in this chapter.

Posttraumatic stress symptoms

While PTSD is somewhat of a catch-all label for trauma-related disorders in colloquial language, it is not the only diagnosis relevant to youth MVC survivors. There are distinctions between PTSD and similar diagnoses that are worthy of consideration among non-clinical parties. Familiarity with these nuanced, yet significant, differences can assist educators in symptom conceptualization and response planning.

In the event that full PTSD diagnostic criteria are not fulfilled, a label of posttraumatic stress symptoms (PTSS) may be considered for individuals who report at least one symptom from each PTSD symptom cluster. However, PTSS is not recognized in the *Diagnostic and statistical manual of mental health disorders* (DSM-5), thus subthreshold PTSD symptoms may be overlooked when a "full" diagnosis is not given.

In the absence of PTSD diagnoses, PTSS that is sufficient to inhibit children's functionality at school may still be present. One study found that about 50% of children were reported by a parent to experience at least minimal impairment from PTSS after the collision. In 9% of cases that did not meet full PTSD diagnostic criteria, parents described their children's symptoms as "extremely problematic" (9). One must consider how simply the perception of such incapacitating PTSS could have anything but deleterious effects on children's learning capacity. While it may be a worthwhile endeavor to confirm the veracity of parents' ratings using additional data sources (i.e., self and teacher reports), at least minimal impairments in academic functioning following involvement in a MVC can be anticipated. To be sure, sub-threshold PTSD is not indicative of the absence of symptoms potentially detrimental to children's success in school settings.

The prevalence rates for PTSD and PTSS are highly comparable. The incidence of PTSS closely mirrored that of PTSD, at approximately 30% of youth survivors one month after the collision. This number subsequently declined to roughly 13% three to six months post-collision (9).

Acute stress disorder

There is an additional disorder worthy of consideration by educators for its relevance to the time after which children involved in MVCs may return to school. To be diagnosed with PTSD, an individual must experience symptoms for at least one month. Therefore, it is not possible for individuals to be diagnosed with PTSD within the initial month following their collision. Instead, a diagnosis of acute stress disorder (ASD) may be given to individuals who experience stress-related symptoms within 3 days to one month post-collision (11).

The prevalence rate of ASD following a traumatic injury was 10% in one sample of children. Twenty-five percent of these children were subsequently diagnosed with PTSD (12). Prevalence rates differ greatly across studies however, with some reporting diagnosable PTSD in 75% of individuals who were first diagnosed with ASD (12). Although children who return to school within one month of their collision cannot, by definition, be diagnosed with PTSD, they may experience trauma-related symptoms. Moreover, they may be diagnosed with ASD and they may already have returned to classrooms.

Posttraumatic stress disorder with delayed expression

It is also possible for trauma-related symptom onset to be delayed at least six months. In this case, neither ASD nor PTSD would be diagnosable within the initial six months following the collision because symptoms are not yet present. When the onset of symptoms sufficient to warrant a PTSD diagnosis occurs at least six months after the traumatic event, a diagnosis of posttraumatic stress disorder with delayed expression (PTSD-DE) may be considered (11). PTSD-DE was found in 25% of youth traffic collision survivors (i.e., age 6-20 years) 18 months following the collision. These children were given doubtful or mild PTSD ratings at 2-16 days post-collision and again at 12-15 weeks post-collision (13). This finding demonstrates the potential for stress-related symptoms to appear long after recovery from physical injury has commenced and the child has returned to school.

Irrespective of diagnosable PTSD or related disorders, 42% of children endorsed adverse psychological reactions 18-months post-collision, and 39% of parents reported negative changes in their child's behavior at school (13). The most commonly reported behavior problems included frequent arguing, excessive talking, day dreaming, restlessness, temper tantrums, and poor concentration. Educators may wish to conceptualize these behaviors as stemming from exposure to traumatic events, especially if a MVC history is known, to avoid mistakenly attributing behaviors to subsidiary causes. Even if children have no trauma-related diagnosis of any kind, there may still be residual effects that can influence their presentation at school.

Comorbidity

The job of educators and mental health professionals is complicated by high comorbidity among trauma disorders and other mental health conditions including depression and anxiety (14), and attention-deficit hyperactivity disorder (ADHD) (5). If, for example, restlessness or poor concentration is exhibited in the classroom post-MVC, these behaviors may be erroneously designated as ADHD, when in reality they could be unrelated to the neurodevelopmental disorder. For children with premorbid ADHD symptomatology, dual diagnoses may be appropriate, and children's extant attentional issues may worsen following exposure to a traumatic event.

In addition to ADHD, youth MVC survivors may also develop clinically significant levels of depression and anxiety. These symptoms may present concurrently with PTSD symptoms, or children may be diagnosed with these disorders instead of PTSD (14). Because multiple diagnoses share behavioral profiles, careful consideration of etiology is required. It is possible that trauma survivors are currently in classrooms with these comorbid diagnoses, for whom histories of trauma exposure have not yet been discovered.

Summary of trauma-related disorders

The onset and severity of stress-related symptomatology may vary widely across youth survivors of motor vehicle collisions. Because diagnosable symptom onset may occur as soon as three days post-collision or be delayed for at least six months, it is necessary for educators to continually monitor collision survivors for symptom development. Teachers may be particularly useful in monitoring symptoms given their frequent interaction with and observation of the children in their classrooms. Familiarity with common MVC-related symptom profiles may aid educators in recognizing trauma-related symptoms in children whose collision histories are both known and unknown.

Teachers may wish to monitor collision survivors for the behavior changes mentioned above, which could indicate the onset of symptoms or an increase in symptom severity. For example, if a child returns to school within six months of their collision, they may initially appear to be functioning at premorbid levels, only to then develop PTSD-DE within a few weeks or months. Conversely, symptoms may appear relatively quickly (i.e., within days of the collision) before the individual has been formally evaluated. Here, immediate classroom accommodations may be necessary and appropriate despite the absence of a formal diagnosis. In any case (i.e., ASD, PTSD, or PTSD-DE), immediate and prolonged monitoring of symptoms is essential to recognizing children in need of care.

Educators are well-suited to monitor their students in conjunction with regular mental health evaluations to assess symptomatology, provide diagnostic clarity, and specify treatment recommendations. Monitoring and evaluating collision survivors' symptoms is crucial because teachers' reports of student behavior often provide invaluable data during an evaluation. Moreover, the provision of necessary and appropriate services, such as classroom accommodations, may be contingent on diagnoses from mental health professionals. The resultant trauma-related diagnoses may aid educators in their conceptualizations of survivors' problematic behavior, the etiology of which could be trauma.

CORRELATES OF TRAUMA DISORDERS

Beyond the symptom profiles and diagnostic criteria of trauma-related disorders, research has identified signs, or correlates, of these disorders that may assist teachers in identifying children in need of care. First, the literature indicates that all children involved in MVCs are at risk for developing PTSD, regardless of the type of collision (i.e., motor vehicle occupant, pedestrian, bicyclist) (10). Furthermore, PTSD is not limited only to children who suffer severe physical injuries. In a review of eight studies assessing the link between physical injury severity and PTSD symptomatology in youth collision survivors (9), only one study found a significant positive relationship (8). The review suggests that more traumatic collisions, as measured by the degree of physical injury suffered, are not predictive of greater PTSD responses among children.

It is therefore important that educators avoid overlooking students who are physically unscathed, for they may be experiencing significant psychological maladjustment that is relatively invisible. Additionally, the degree of physical injury sustained cannot reliably be used to triage survivors for the provision of psychological services, as well as the implementation of classroom accommodations. Put simply, the absence of or recovery from physical injury does not mean the child has returned to premorbid functioning. There may still be emotional and psychological consequences that inhibit children's academic performance. Schools and mental health professionals will best serve MVC survivors when alternative means are used to assess the urgency and appropriateness of intervention.

Peritraumatic distress

More important than physical injury is the child's perceived level of threat (10) and the intensity of distress (9) during or immediately following the collision, known as peritraumatic distress. Peritraumatic distress has been shown to strongly predict the presence of PTSD symptoms in children five weeks after their collisions (15). For example, children who were involved in fatal MVCs reported more PTSD symptoms than children involved in collisions in which everyone survived (16).

High peritraumatic distress is therefore a sign of children at risk for PTSD. In the event that a child returns to school within a few weeks of their collision, effective symptom monitoring may include probing for signs of peritraumatic distress via direct and indirect assessment. If the child is developmentally capable of the language and emotion necessary to effectively recall and process a traumatic event, a direct approach may be appropriate and useful. Here, educators may listen for indications of fear or helplessness during or immediately following the collision. For younger children, insight into their experiences may be accessible indirectly, through play or other less potentially harmful approaches.

In addition to developmental stage, appropriate inquiry regarding peritraumatic distress depends on children's perceptions of safety in their school environments. The degree to which children endorse presently feeling safe at school may be indicative of their readiness to reflect on peritraumatic experiences. Furthermore, survivors of trauma often express concern about the safety of their family members (5). Teachers can also ask children about their loved ones, which may be welcomed as a gesture of care and support. Prior to their assessment of peritraumatic experiences, however, it is worthwhile for teachers to reassure children that not only are they now safe, but their family members are safe as well.

Although useful in screening children at risk for symptoms of trauma, assessing peritraumatic distress should be done with caution. Assessment should not occur prematurely or too directly, risking the re-exposure of children to traumatic stimuli. In other words, care must be taken not to induce painful memories of the collision, which likely will reduce children's perceptions of comfort and safety at school. The student-teacher relationship may also be compromised, as the teacher becomes associated with threatening reminders of traumatic events. There is a fine line between effective risk assessment and overwhelming children by encouraging too much reflection, too soon, especially if the children are hypervigilant in detecting threats to safety (5). To minimize the risk of re-traumatization, effective collaboration between caregivers, educators, and mental health professionals will aid in the assessment of peritraumatic distress to more accurately predict susceptibility to PTSD.

Trauma history

Children's trauma histories are also important to consider when assessing risk for PTSD following a MVC. The relationship between trauma history and PTSD remains equivocal however, and is perhaps dependent on the nature of the traumatic experience (i.e., whether the child was involved in a MVC or experienced a traumatic event of another type). For example, previous involvement in MVCs was shown to predict fewer PTSD symptoms in children following subsequent MVCs (8). Such a finding suggests that children may become desensitized to the perception that their lives are threatened, having previously survived at least one collision. As has been shown, reduced threat perceptions (i.e., peritraumatic distress) during a collision subsequently reduce one's risk for PTSD.

Conversely, repeated exposure to traumatic events other than MVCs has been linked to increased prevalence of PTSD in children involved in MVCs. A traumatic experience within 12 months prior to the collision significantly predicted the presence of PTSD symptoms (10). Children who experience distress from non-MVC related events also endorse PTSD symptoms at a higher rate (16). It is therefore plausible that desensitization to peritraumatic distress may be limited to the milieu of collision-related trauma.

This is an important point for educators who may be familiar with additional stressors in a child's environment, such as histories of abuse or the witnessing of domestic violence. Non-MVC-related stressors that are either greater in number or in severity may make a seemingly innocuous MVC, when viewed in isolation, increasingly more problematic. More holistic approaches to symptom prediction may indeed be more accurate.

Social support

What has been presented heretofore is a tripartite model (i.e., physical injury, peritraumatic distress, and trauma history) for predicting the onset and severity of PTSD symptoms among child collision survivors. Familiarity with the correlates of MVC-related PTSD may enable educators to more robustly predict or identify manifestations of PTSD in the classroom, and then allocate resources accordingly. The applicability of any one correlate to a specific child may be determined through direct observation in the classroom, or by carefully crafting probing questions consistent with the child's developmental level. Additional sources of information include parents and mental health professionals. Assessing any one of these risk factors can be done in a way that causes children to feel supported by caring individuals, which serves as a protective factor against trauma symptoms, depression, and anger (8).

Providing children with immediate social support following their collision has been shown to decrease subsequent avoidance behaviors: a primary symptom of PTSD (8). Although educators are unlikely to intervene immediately following a collision, they can provide children with continued social support upon their return to school. Students can be provided opportunities to speak to supportive adults when they need a reprieve from scheduled activities. This is especially effective when planned in advanced, such that meetings become routine and predictable (5). By fostering an environment in which children are comfortable processing their traumatic experiences, by talking and thinking about the event, educators may be viewed as allies in their recovery. Research shows that adults who assist children in processing their traumatic experiences and reassure positive outcomes are considered most supportive by youth trauma survivors (8).

Providing children with supportive experiences is crucial to recovery when you consider the plasticity of a developing brain. Children's brains are adaptable, meaning the effects of traumatic experiences can be mitigated under appropriate conditions: effective intervention in a supportive environment (5).

Providing social support not only safeguards children from PTSD symptoms, it is useful in garnering information pertinent to each risk factor in the tripartite model.

IMPACT ON LEARNING

One out of every four children has experienced trauma that can impact their learning and behavior in school (17). Thus far, the focus of this chapter has been to describe trauma-related disorders that may occur in children following their involvement in a MVC. I also presented empirically supported correlates, or factors associated with trauma, that may prove useful to educators in identifying children who are at risk for developing a trauma-related disorder. In short, I attempted to answer the following questions; What are the signs and symptoms of trauma-related disorders, and when might it be useful for educators to consider exposure to trauma as the origin of children's behavior in the classroom? With this knowledge in mind, I now turn to a discussion of how trauma-related symptoms may manifest in children at school, and address how school systems can respond.

In the sections that follow, I review the impact of MVC-related trauma on children's ability to learn and perform in academic settings. I begin by describing how patterns of student behavior and teacher response are context specific, and depend on the nature of their specific interaction. Next, I discuss how trauma is related to intellectual functioning. Specifically, I provide evidence for the detrimental effects of trauma on children's performance in the verbal domain, and discuss direct implications for functional enhancement. Then, I introduce changes in behavior patterns and cognitive profiles that are associated with involvement in MVCs among children. Later, I discuss the role of parents in the recovery process and explain how their involvement can be managed effectively. Finally, I conclude with a discussion of implications for educators, as well as a review of strategies that schools can implement to maximize students' success following a MVC.

The teacher-student dyad

There are three bipolar, interrelated dimensions that must be considered when describing how trauma impacts children's behavior in classrooms. These factors are also likely to shape educators' responses to children's behavior.

That is, the nature and degree of response are contingent on the characteristics of each teacher-student dyad as defined by three factors. First, teachers' responses may be dependent on whether children's trauma histories are known or unknown. If a child's trauma history is known, teachers may be more likely to respond in ways that are sensitive to children's experiences of trauma. If trauma histories are unknown or are not ruled-out as roots of behavior, traumatized children and their behaviors can be profoundly misunderstood (5).

For example, when they do not follow teachers' instructions, teachers may conclude that children are simply being defiant and choosing to disobey, which is likely to be frustrating to teachers and disruptive to the learning environment. This sequence perpetuates the erroneous conclusion of "difficult" children. As will be shown, this conclusion is often inaccurate. It may be that these children's unique needs and challenges are overlooked and misunderstood, resulting in a greater likelihood of punitive rather than trauma-sensitive action. If thought to be "problem-children," these students and their behaviors can strain teacher-student relationships over time, moving them ever-closer to falling behind their peers.

Second, the perceptibility of students' behaviors may differ depending on whether the teacher-student dyads are working directly or indirectly, which can be thought of as variable along a continuum. Direct interaction, in this sense, refers to the proximity of teachers to students, either in terms of physical distance or by the level of attention given to students by teachers. The outcome of the interaction is also important to consider in determining its location along this continuum. Direct interaction may increase the likelihood that trauma-related behaviors (or symptoms), when present, are observable and correctly identified by teachers.

Conversely, indirect interaction refers to proximity or attention that causes behaviors to go unnoticed. In this case, the behaviors may be inconspicuous to educators whose attention is divided among numerous students in the classroom. Even if teachers become aware of the behaviors, they are likely to be misidentified or their cause may be misattributed to something other than trauma exposure. Indirect interaction is increasingly likely in schools with larger class sizes and limited resources, wherein children with trauma-related disorders could go unnoticed.

Third, regardless of whether children's trauma histories are known, teachers may respond to students' behaviors differently when they are conceptualized as symptoms of trauma-related disorders. The conceptualization may or may not be correct. If not, behaviors that are manifestations of trauma-symptoms are erroneously attributed to a secondary cause (e.g., a mood disorder). Ideally, children's trauma histories will be known to educators, increasing the likelihood that trauma-related behaviors are properly identified and teachers' responses are trauma-sensitive.

Verbal skills

One key area in which childhood trauma can have deleterious effects on academic achievement is language and communication skills. Trauma, or more specifically the hypervigilance associated with trauma, deactivates areas of the brain that are required for academic learning. The regions of the brain that operate during fearful states override areas of the brain that are active when learning (18). As a result, traumatized children who exhibit persistent hypervigilance or who do not feel safe at school may show deficits in the ability to learn, perceive, and express verbal information (5). These tasks require activation of brain regions in the left hemisphere. Conversely, hyperarousal of the right hemisphere during hypervigilance allocates the brain's energy for emotional and sensory processing, thereby deactivating areas used in verbal processing and communication.

Children who are less able to perceive and express language may therefore be unable to respond appropriately to verbal instructions from teachers. These deficits may be obvious to teachers who are working directly with students if they are immediately noncompliant when given verbal instructions. Two responses from the teacher are plausible in this situation, depending on the teacher's knowledge of trauma-related symptoms and behaviors. First, the teacher may conclude that the student has deficits in verbal comprehension, perhaps due to hypervigilance from trauma exposure, which has caused a misperception or misunderstanding of the instructions. A trauma-sensitive response would be one in which the teacher then repeats, rephrases, or shortens the directions to facilitate the child's understanding. If in this case exposure to trauma is not considered or is dismissed, the teacher could erroneously conclude that the student is making a conscious decision to disobey the instructions. Here, teachers may perceive students' behaviors as acts of defiance and become frustrated by noncompliance. Discipline then becomes a likely course of action.

Intellectual functioning

There is evidence for diminished capacity in the verbal domain among traumatized children according to their performance on intellectual assessments. Children diagnosed with PTSD perform significantly lower on verbal intelligence measures than children without PTSD, regardless of both the time since exposure and the child's developmental level at the time of exposure (19). This means that trauma exposure at any stage of childhood can have damaging effects on cognitive development long after the exposure occurred.

The cognitive capacities that are assessed by verbal domain tasks on the *Wechsler Intelligence Scales* include auditory discrimination, auditory comprehension, auditory processing speed and expressive language (20). Deficiencies in any of these areas can inhibit children's abilities to communicate effectively with teachers and peers. Children with PTSD also scored significantly lower on a global measure of intelligence than children without PTSD, although their performance may have been heavily influenced by relatively poor performance on verbal tasks (19). Still, the cause for concern is the evidence that supports the positive association between intellectual functioning and academic achievement. Verbal comprehension abilities and global intelligence are highly correlated with academic achievement, at .80 and .87, respectively (20). In other words, assessments of intelligence and academic achievement measure at least 80% of the same abilities. Therefore, students with PTSD whose verbal skills are diminished are less likely to achieve academic success.

POSTTRAUMATIC STRESS IN THE CLASSROOM

In this section I discuss cognitive profiles and behavioral patterns that are common among youth MVC survivors. One way to classify trauma response is along a continuum from adaptive to maladaptive, or in the case of schools, from school-appropriate to school-inappropriate behavior. I contend that the opposite poles of this continuum are problematic in certain situations or contexts. While the semantics are probably less important to the big picture, it is important to consider the dualistic nature (i.e., adaptive or maladaptive) of each cognitive profile and behavioral pattern. I refer to dualism, in this case, as thoughts and behaviors that can be either helpful or harmful.

Consider hyperarousal, for example. Hyperarousal is considered a symptom of PTSD; thus, it is inherently characteristic of a disorder. Herein lies the problem. On one hand, hyperarousal may be problematic in a classroom and efforts may be taken to suppress manifestations of the symptom. Children may be required to sit in their seat quietly or face a consequence. In this context hyperarousal has a negative connotation. On the other hand, hyperarousal is useful in detecting threat for the sake of avoiding danger and preserving safety. For an individual who has experienced trauma, sensing and avoiding danger may be a quite welcomed "symptom." In fact, efforts to suppress hyperarousal could be threatening to the individual. Therefore, it may instead be more appropriate to conceptualize trauma responses along a continuum from distressing to fulfilling, noting the dualism of any one response style.

The cognitive profiles to which I refer are drawn from a posttraumatic response model developed by Tedeschi, Park, and Calhoun in 1998 (7). They reflect changes in children's philosophies on life as well as the meaning and significance ascribed to social relationships. The behavioral patterns correspond to and are indicative of these cognitive changes that many children undergo following their MVCs. As mentioned, both thoughts and behaviors can be conducive or disruptive to children's learning.

External locus of control

With respect to cognitions, many children involved in MVCs believe that future events are largely outside of their control (21). This belief reflects a deterministic worldview that stands in contrast to the notion of "free will" (22). Deterministic cognitions may result from the perception that they were not at fault for their collision, and yet the collision occurred. Furthermore, they may believe that their involvement in the MVC was unavoidable and thus their experiences with fate are generalized to other areas of life (i.e., outside of the transportation milieu).

An external locus of control is problematic though, because it renders children unable to identify causal relationships between their behavior and the events in their lives (5). When the link between behavior and consequence is ambiguous, children may then adopt a laissez-faire attitude, become passive, aloof or withdrawn, and engage in riskier behavior. Each of these responses reflect an internalized, deterministic relationship between actions and outcomes. By adopting this way of thinking, school children may lack motivation on academic tasks (5) and in other areas in which persistence is associated with mastery.

Perception on life

Children who are involved in MVCs may alter their perceptions on the value and meaning of life, as well as modify how they navigate their environment. Traumatized children are likely to perceive life as fragile and infallible, and themselves as vulnerable (21). They understand that life is finite and cannot be taken for granted. In this mindset, children may take excessive precautions to ensure their safety and the safety of others, both in transportation contexts and beyond. This response may be driven by fear of repeated physical or psychological injury. Insecurity may surround the realization that life can be dangerous and that safety is not guaranteed. Children may avoid situations in which even the slightest potential threat is present. No longer are they able to bask in blissful ignorance or youthful naiveté, which can lead them to be unduly fearful of danger in their environment.

Changes in perception can also engender an adaptive behavioral response, causing children to prepare to navigate potential threats to which they may regularly be exposed (e.g., crossing a busy street). By successfully managing environmental threats, children may ultimately feel capable of preserving their safety, leading them to a newfound sense of self-sustainability. Children involved in MVCs also experience a heightened appreciation for life (21). A "live life to the fullest" mentality may motivate an individual to engage in meaningful activities before opportunities pass. These activities, such as spending time with loved ones, are prioritized and concurrently become more enjoyable (21). In summary, changes in perceptions of life can lead children to be fearful of threats in their environment and become inhibited, or they can embrace the need to protect themselves and their loved ones from ever-present danger.

Relationships

When children return to school following their MVC, they are reintroduced to the classroom's social system. As a result, elements of that system (i.e., the students in the classroom) undergo adjustment, most notably in the way that other students respond to MVC survivors. Some children report improved peer relationships at school following their MVC, such that they gained popularity or determined who would reliably support them in times of need (21). Increased popularity is a potential secondary gain and may incentivize children to share their collision experience with their peers. If done so in a way that communicates a disturbance (e.g., pain or worry), this behavior could imitate re-experiencing symptoms that are characteristic of trauma-related disorders. Teachers are encouraged to consider children's motivations for sharing their stories, and differentiate genuine descriptions of peritraumatic distress from sensationalized details for the purpose of story enhancement.

Many children also reported that their relationships with others deteriorated, especially when support was expected but not provided (21). Social support is not only beneficial in decreasing avoidance behaviors, it also affirms for children the types of trusting relationships that they believe have been established.

Parental involvement

The development of PTSD is not limited solely to individuals directly involved in a MVC. Parents of MVC survivors can develop PTSD either by witnessing the collision directly or by learning that their child was involved. In a sample of parental witnesses, the prevalence of PTSD for parents was comparable to that of child survivors (23). This suggests that as MVCs are perceived as more traumatic to children, they will also elicit more trauma-related responses in parents. As the experience of distress increases, the onset of PTSD becomes more likely in both parties.

Like children re-entering the classroom, parent and child relationships also undergo change following a collision. Many children report that their parents now express more worry about them and more closely monitor their activities (8). For educators, this could mean regular contact with parents, who are eager to ensure their children's safety when outside of their supervision. Parents may go as far as to express distrust in the school's capacity to safeguard their children. They may ultimately take matters into their own hands, for example, by no longer allowing their children to ride the bus, and choosing instead to pick them up from school. What can be perceived as parental hypervigilance, or "helicopter parenting," may be disconcerting to educators. Further, while it may be well-intentioned, parental involvement may worsen children's experiences at school. It is important for educators not to ignore parental (hyper) vigilance, however. Research suggests that parental vigilance is positively correlated with children's PTSD symptoms (8). Increased parental involvement is yet another signal of children who are potentially in need of more immediate or intensive care.

Educators can also be cognizant of disruption in the family system (i.e., altered relationships) and the family environment (i.e., living spaces). Following a MVC, some parents report financial loss, disruption of employment, and discord among spouses (8). Educators can anticipate a period of instability in children's lives, which could have myriad effects on school performance. In fact, classrooms may represent the only normalcy, stability, or predictability for these children. A predictable school environment may mitigate the effects of family instability. To enhance predictability, it is important for children to establish routines and for schools to provide additional support when disruptions in routines are anticipated.

Parents and help-seeking

In a study of MVC-PTSD among parent and child survivors (23), less than half of parents sought any type of professional help for their children, despite the presence of symptoms sufficient to warrant a diagnosis of PTSD. Incidentally, only 20% of parents sought treatment for themselves. It is evident that mental health services are heavily underutilized by child MVC survivors and their families. Educators cannot assume that children are receiving treatment even when symptoms are sufficiently severe to warrant a trauma disorder diagnosis. Here is an opportunity for educators to potentially influence whether treatment is sought.

First, because teachers regularly interact with students, they can monitor children for signs and symptoms of trauma. Of course, monitoring will be most effective when teachers are trained to look in the right places. Second, it has been shown that parental involvement is likely to increase, providing teachers with opportunities to offer social support to parents in ways that are effective with traumatized children. If more members of the family feel supported by the school, perhaps they will be more receptive to the idea of seeking help.

Posttraumatic behavior change

Traumatized children often exhibit a variety of behaviors in the classroom that can cue observers to properly identify behavior as manifestations of trauma-related symptomatology. It is important to consider that the behavioral manifestations of trauma occur along a continuum, from internal to external presentations (5). Educators are encouraged to be mindful of children who express their symptoms outwardly, as well as children for whom social withdrawal renders symptom identification more ambiguous. The degree to which behavioral changes are present will necessarily depend on children's premorbid patterns of behavior. For example, for a child who exhibits premorbid hyperactivity, manifestations of PTSD-hyperarousal symptoms may be less noticeable. Conversely, for a child with premorbid inattentive tendencies, day-dreaming will appear less symptomatic. Ambiguity around behavior change may lead to the conclusion that trauma-related symptoms are absent.

The *National Child Traumatic Stress Network* provides a toolkit for educators that enumerates common symptomatology in children and adolescents (17). The following is a summary of its inclusions. Most notably, traumatized children's development may stagnate or regress across numerous dimensions, which highlights the need for immediate and appropriate intervention. Next, traumatized children are often resistant to transitions or unexpected changes in their routines. A lack of structure and predictability may be the cause of mood swings and temper tantrums that are commonly observed among these children (13).

Impairments in attention and concentration are also characteristic of trauma exposure, as are memory and problem solving issues. Children can be irritable, impulsive, and hyperactive, or they may withdraw socially and appear aloof. Furthermore, these children are likely to worry more about their safety and the safety of others around them. The result is reluctance to engage in behavior that is deemed too threatening, which is applicable even to activities that were considered innocuous prior to the collision.

Many traumatized children also engage in collision-related play, while others will demonstrate new fears of transportation related toys (e.g., bicycles). Somatic complaints are also common, which may or may not be related to physical pain from an injury suffered during the collision. These complaints may include headaches or stomach aches, for example, for which there is often no identifiable organic or neurologic basis (24). Disturbances in sleep and appetite patterns may also be reported. With regard to arousal, children often overreact or underreact to unexpected sounds or movement in their environment (e.g., schedule bells or closing locker doors). They are also likely to exhibit anxiety around separation from parents and teachers (17).

CONCLUSION: IMPLICATIONS FOR EDUCATORS

The relationship between educators and trauma-related symptomatology can be conceptualized in three dimensions: observation, identification or attribution, and response. The first step is being able to observe behavior that is associated with exposure to trauma. One might ask, is the teacher aware of a child's behavior that may or may not be trauma-related? Second, the behavior is differentiated from behaviors unrelated to trauma. The question becomes, can the teacher, in collaboration with a team of caregivers, properly identify trauma as the root cause of particular behaviors? Third, assuming the answer to these questions is yes, the final step is to respond appropriately. Is the teacher's response trauma-sensitive, or is it punitive? Trauma survivors will be best served in environments where these questions can be answered in the affirmative.

To the degree that children subjectively perceive current threats in their environment, symptoms of trauma persist (25). First and foremost, it is critical that children perceive emotional and physical safety at school for learning and development to occur (5). Perceptions of safety can be enhanced when triggers, or reminders of the traumatic event, are removed from the environment. For example, teachers may wish to remove students prior to fire drills, or when police officers or firefighters visit the school. While teachers and school administrators play an important role in physically securing classrooms (e.g., by locking doors), children's subjective appraisal of security in the environment must also be addressed (26). In doing so, it is important to remember that what may feel safe and secure to non-traumatized children may be perceived as threatening to trauma survivors (5).

By becoming familiar with the signs and symptoms of trauma, teachers are better equipped to respond appropriately to the unique needs of traumatized children in their classrooms. Increasing knowledge of trauma-related disorders may also serve to lessen teachers' anxiety or apprehension when confronted with unusual or challenging behavior, by guiding their response.

However, it is important to note that classroom teachers may have limited training in trauma assessment and intervention. They are not therapists and thus the responsibility of identifying and caring for traumatized children should not fall solely onto their shoulders. A collaborative system of care is essential, wherein educators serve as important links between trauma survivors, their families, and mental health professionals. Collaboration may also involve the school nurse, school psychologist, school administrators, and any other party enlisted by the family to participate in their child's care.

It has been suggested that teachers develop a supportive relationship with trauma survivors in which children are comfortable talking about their experiences. Over the course of these discussions, the potential exists for teachers to be exposed to content that is deeply disturbing, leaving them vulnerable to vicarious traumatization. The adage states, "you cannot help others without first helping yourself."

Teachers are encouraged to consider their readiness to provide support, especially when they have trauma histories of their own. If they are uncomfortable, feel overwhelmed, or are unable to meet the needs of their students, they must seek assistance. Support may be provided by administrators, colleagues, or individuals outside of the school system, such as family and friends or professional counselors. Support and guidance is essential, not only for traumatized children, but for individuals responsible for their care. Effective collaboration and help-seeking will protect educators from vicarious victimization and burnout, and enhance the educational experience for survivors of trauma.

REFERENCES

[1]   Centers for Disease Control and Prevention. Injury prevention and control. Web-based injury statistics query and reporting system; 2014. URL: https://www.cdc.gov/injury/wisqars/index.html.
[2]   US Department of Transportation, National Highway Traffic Safety Administration. Motor vehicle traffic crashes as a leading cause of death in the United States, 2012-2014. URL: https://crashstats.nhtsa.dot.gov/Api/Public/ViewPublication/812297.
[3]   Centers for Disease Control and Prevention. Nonfatal injury data. Leading causes of nonfatal injury reports, 2013. URL: http://webappa.cdc.gov/sasweb/ncipc/nfilead2000.html.
[4]   National Center for Education Statistics. Schools and staffing survey. Average number of hours in the school day and average number of days in the school year for public schools, by state: 2007-08. URL: https://nces.ed.gov/surveys/sass/tables/sass0708_035_s1s.asp.

[5] Cole SF, Greenwald J, Gadd MG, Ristuccia J, Wallace DL, Gregory M. Helping traumatized children learn, 6th ed. URL: https://traumasensitiveschools.org/tlpi-publications/download-a-free-copy-of-helping-traumatized-children-learn/.
[6] Posttraumatic stress disorder. American Psychiatric Association, 2013. URL: http://www.dsm5.org/Documents/PTSD%20Fact%20Sheet.pdf.
[7] Tedeschi RG, Park CL, Calhoun, LG. Posttraumatic growth: Positive changes in the aftermath of crisis. Mahwah, NJ: Erlbaum, 1998:203-12.
[8] Keppel-Benson JM, Ollendick TH, Benson MJ. Post-traumatic stress in children following motor vehicle accidents. J Child Psychol Psychiatry 2002;43(2):203-12.
[9] Olofsson E, Bunketorp O, Andersson AL. Children and adolescents injured in traffic -associated psychological consequences: a literature review. Acta Paediatrica 2009;98(1): 17-22.
[10] Stallard P, Velleman R, Baldwin S. Prospective study of post-traumatic stress disorder in children involved in road traffic accidents. BMJ 1998;317(7173):1619-23.
[11] American Psychiatric Association. Diagnostic and statistical manual of mental disorders, (DSM-V). 5th ed. Washington, DC: American Psychiatric Association; 2015.
[12] Bryant RA, Salmon K, Sinclair E, Davidson P. The relationship between acute stress disorder and posttraumatic stress disorder in injured children. J Traumatic Stress 2007;20(6):1075-9.
[13] Gillies ML, Barton J, Di GA. Follow-up of young road accident victims. J Traumatic Stress 2003;16(5):523-6.
[14] Stallard P, Velleman R, Langsford J, Baldwin S. Coping and psychological distress in children involved in road traffic accidents. Br J Clin Psychol 2001;40:197-208.
[15] Bui E, Brunet A, Allenou C, Camassel C, Raynaud JP, Claudet I, et al. Peritraumatic reactions and posttraumatic stress symptoms in school-aged children victims of road traffic accident. Gen Hosp Psychiatry 2010;32(3):321-7.
[16] Tierens M, Bal S, Crombez, G, Van VP, Rosseel Y, Antrop I, et al. The traumatic impact of motor vehicle accidents in high school students. J Pediatr Psychol 2012;37:1-6.
[17] The National Child Traumatic Stress Network (2008). Child trauma toolkit for educators. URL: http://nctsn.org/sites/default/files/assets/pdfs/Child_Trauma_ Toolkit_Final.pdf.
[18] Perry BD. Neurodevelopmental impact of violence in childhood. In: Schetky DH, Benedek EP, eds. Principles and practice of child and adolescent forensic psychiatry. Washington, DC: American Psychiatric Publishing, 2002:191-203.
[19] Saigh PA, Yasik AE, Oberfield RA, Halamandaris PV, Bremner JD. The intellectual performance of traumatized children and adolescents with or without posttraumatic stress disorder. J Abnorm Psychol 2006;115(2):332-40.
[20] Lichtenberger EO, Kaufman AS. Essentials of WAIS-IV assessment. Hoboken, NJ: John Wiley, 2013.
[21] Salter E, Stallard P. Posttraumatic growth in child survivors of a road traffic accident. J Traumatic Stress 2004;17(4):335-40.

[22] Cervone D, Pervin LA. Personality: theory and research. Hoboken, NJ: John Wiley, 2013.
[23] de Vries APJ, Kassam-Adams N, Cnaan A, Sherman-Slate E, Gallagher PR, Winston FK. Looking beyond the physical injury: posttraumatic stress disorder in children and parents after pediatric traffic injury. Pediatrics 1999;104(6):1293-9.
[24] Asmundson GJ, Thibodeau MA, Peluso DL. Somatoform disorders. In: Herson M, Beidel DC, eds. Adult psychopathology and diagnosis. Hoboken, NJ: John Wiley, 2012:471-95.
[25] Ehlers A, Clark DM. A cognitive model of post-traumatic stress disorder. Behav Res Ther 2000;38:319-45.
[26] Stallard P, Smith E. Appraisals and cognitive coping styles associated with chronic post-traumatic symptoms in child road traffic accident survivors. J Child Psychol Psychiatry 2007;48(2):194-201.

In: Children and Youth
Editors: Donald E. Greydanus et al.
ISBN: 978-1-53611-102-6
© 2017 Nova Science Publishers, Inc.

Chapter 9

RESILIENCE IN YOUTH AFTER MOTOR VEHICLE ACCIDENTS

Mark S Barajas[*], PhD and Heath Schechinger, PhD

Department of Psychology, School of Science,
Saint Mary's College of California, Moraga, California, US
Counseling and Psychological Services, University of California Berkeley,
Berkeley, California, US

Resilience is generally understood as the ability to bounce back from setbacks and overcome adversity. Considering children and adolescents, although up to 40% of youth involved in motor accidents develop symptoms of post-traumatic stress disorder (PTSD), the majority do not. What differentiates the young people who remain mostly symptom free from those who develop PTSD? How can medical professionals help to promote resilience among youth involved in motor vehicle accidents? This review provides an overview of resilience by defining key terms, summarizing nearly fifty years of research, explaining current models of resilience, and suggesting interventions intended to enhance and support resiliency among youth involved in motor vehicle accidents.

Keywords: Resilience, empathy, strength-based, active listening, hope

---

[*] Correspondence: Assistant professor Mark S Barajas, PhD, Department of Psychology, School of Science, Saint Mary's College of California, 1928 St Mary's Road, Moraga, CA 94575, United States. Email: mb37@stmarys-ca.edu.

INTRODUCTION

Over 400,000 children and adolescents experience motor vehicle accidents ever year in the United States and research suggests between 14 and 40% of them will develop post-traumatic stress disorder (PTSD) (1, 2). Perhaps surprisingly, injury severity is a poor predictor of PTSD symptoms. In contrast, cognitive factors such as the meaning an accident victim ascribes to the event, the emotional coping strategies used, and the perception of the accident's threat are much stronger predictors of developing PTSD (3). Thus, cognitive factors, along with social supports, are understood to be indicators of resilience, providing the foundation for those children and adolescents who cope with being involved in a motor vehicle accident without developing PTSD. The following chapter explores the past five decades of research on resilience, highlighting factors and models for conceptualizing resilience, as well as interventions for working with children who may be at risk of developing PTSD following a motor vehicle accident.

What is resilience?

The concept of resilience is often cited when attempting to explain potential responses to challenging or traumatic events. A child responding "favorably" to a difficult situation is often thought of as being resilient, while a child responding "poorly" might be considered non-resilient. However, defining resilience and describing its development is a complex problem. How resilient an individual is in general and in a given moment is impacted by a number of factors. When considering resilience, it is necessary to consider both the nature of the threat as well as the response to the threat. While certain situations are bound to be perceived as inherently more threatening than others, individual differences in how threatening a certain situation is perceived is going to vary based on an individual's unique genetic disposition (biology), their collective internal experiences (psychology), as well as their environmental factors (socialization). Along with that, what is considered adaptive is largely determined by prevailing cultural expectations.

As resilience continues to be studied across cultures, defining resilience has become increasingly complex because adaptive responses in one culture may not be considered appropriate in another. For example, refusing to leave the house and mourning for a month after the death of a loved one may considered appropriate and adaptive in one culture, and maladaptive in another. Evaluations of 'adaptive' and 'maladaptive' responses can also be assessed in a number of ways, such as in terms of the impact on the community or individual relationships, or by the lack of individual psychopathology following a threatening event. Hence, evaluating resilience is not as simple as it may appear on the surface. In light of all this, we will be adopting Masten's definition, who suggests that resilience is "the capacity of a dynamic system to adapt successfully to disturbances that threaten system function, viability, or development" (4).

KEY CONCEPTS AND TERMS

Accounting for risk factors is a common approach in evaluating resilience. Although certain indicators may suggest heightened risk, they do not guarantee that individuals with those particular risk factors are necessarily going to suffer negative outcomes- hence, it is important to think of risk factors in terms of probabilities. While awareness of discrete risk factors can serve as a helpful heuristic, it can also lead to premature foreclosure. Therefore, each case merits individual consideration, despite the risk factors, as individual patient responses can vary.

There is now considerable evidence to suggest that as risk factors accumulate and persist, resilience decreases and outcomes become less favorable (5, 6). Taking this into consideration, resilience research typically focuses on both the cumulative and individual risk factors. For example, an individual experiencing a new trauma is at greater risk if it is experienced in the context of other ongoing challenges than if it were a single isolated event (7, 8). Furthermore, risk factors and resilience tend to have an inverse relationship- that is, as risk factors increase, resilient responses tend to decline (9).

Predictors of trauma responses are often put into two categories: assets and protective factors. Assets are general resources associated with positive adaptation in common situations, while protective factors are capacities present when experiencing adversity (10). Some factors are generally helpful regardless of the circumstances (e.g., supportive parents, high cognitive functioning), while others are more domain-specific and only helpful in certain circumstances (such as when distress is particularly high or when experiencing a certain type of emergency). Helpful parents, for example, can be helpful by providing day-to-day support as well as support in emergency situations. In contrast, an anxious child may be more likely to experience distress but is also less likely to engage in risky behavior.

Table 1. Wright and Masten's (9) examples of bio-psycho-social-cultural systems and processes potentially implicated in fostering resilience for children and families

Individual Factors	Genetic moderators and epigenetic processes
	Positive physical health and immune function
	Adaptive self-regulation system (physiological, emotional, cognitive, and behavioral)
	Adequacy of stress response systems
	Strong cognitive and problem-solving abilities
	Agency and an effective mastery motivation system
	Adaptive temperament and personality
Family Factors	Close attachment relationships
	Positive extended family and kinship ties
	Cohesiveness, structure, and support within the family
	Effectiveness of parenting in the cultural context
	Family rituals, values, and beliefs
	Financial stability
Community Factors	Safety of the physical environment
	Affordable housing
	Effective education system
	Peer friendships with positive values and norms
	Presence of religious and spiritual communities
	Good public health care and social services
	Employment opportunities
	Adequate access to emergency (police, fire, medical) and legal services
	Access to recreational facilities
Cultural Factors	Belief systems that give life meaning and purpose
	Protective child policies (child labor, child health and welfare policies)
	Socioeconomic policies and health of local and national economy
	Availability and adequacy of emergency response systems
	Access to material resources
	Human rights; Adequacy of general laws and legal systems for protection of citizens
	Prevention of and protection from oppression and political violence
	Global relationships with international community
	Peaceful political situation and some degree of national security

It is not always necessary for researchers to distinguish whether the correlates of resilience are assets or protective factors, because in a number of cases, they could be both. The four most commonly researched correlates of resilience in children include socioeconomic status, relationship with caregivers, schools, and cognitive abilities (10, 11). The available literature clearly suggests that resilient young people are not drawing upon unique or exclusive qualities, but common resources of adaptive capacity within themselves, their interpersonal relationships, and their relationships with other systems (see Table 1 for a list of bio-psycho-social-cultural adaptive systems (9). The following sections summarize the evolution of resiliency research and contemporary understanding of resiliency models.

RESILIENCE RESEARCH AND MODELS

Although an exhaustive review of the construct of resiliency is beyond the scope of this chapter, an overview of resiliency research and contemporary resiliency models is warranted. Readers seeking a more thorough review of resiliency might consider Prince-Embury and Saklofske (12).

Since emerging in the early 1970s, resiliency research has been characterized by four waves of influence (13). The initial motivation for investigating resilience came from scholars who observed positive adaptation and outcomes among groups of children considered to be "at risk" for developing a variety of psychological problems (14). Common to all fields of study, especially those in their early stages, investigators of resilience have at times disagreed on appropriate methods, key concepts, and overarching theoretical conceptualizations of resilience. However, despite these scholarly arguments, the understanding and investigation of resilience has grown more sophisticated and refined over time and has enhanced clinicians' work with children and adolescents.

Wave one: Individual characteristics

The first wave of resiliency research reflected the cultural Zeitgeist of the United States during the 1970s, mostly focusing on individual characteristics, rugged individualism, and a "pull yourself up by your bootstraps" mentality. Children who thrived in the face of adversity were thought to be nearly invulnerable to stress and possess inner strength which functioned as a sort of psychological armor (15, 16).

Thus, scholars produced lists of characteristics, later known as protective factors (e.g., good cognitive abilities, positive outlook, sense of humor) thought to be common in resilient children. Complementing the focus on children's individual traits, other researchers focused on identifying discrete threats to optimal child development and similarly produced lists of elements, later known as risk factors (e.g., poverty, chronic illness, parental divorce). Finally, although many researchers focused on child characteristics, some scholars investigated elements of families, communities, and schools where resilient youth could be found.

Consequently, researchers identified broad correlates (e.g., positive sibling relationships, access to recreational centers, well-trained teachers) situated within particular domains (e.g., family, community, school), which were believed to foster resilience. These early resiliency researchers laid the groundwork for future inquiry by identifying, defining, and categorizing factors associated with resilience.

Wave two: Processes

Complementing the first wave of resiliency research which identified factors associated with resilience, the second wave of scholarship explored processes underlying resilience development. Moreover, second-wave resiliency research explored both pathological and positive outcomes, recognizing resilience as a phenomenon arising from interrelated processes (17, 18). Second-wave researchers sought to illuminate developmental pathways predicting resilience by investigating processes of attachment, moral development, emotional regulation, and motivation. Researchers also began recognizing the influence of culture and more closely investigated family and environmental influences on resilience.

Importantly, second-wave research revealed the development of resilience to be contextual, bidirectional, and impacted by a child's perception of her social context (19). For example, whereas many studies of children at risk found extensive social support predictive of resilience, Cicchetti and Rogosch found maltreated resilient children actually relied on fewer social supports than comparison control subjects (20). Finally, second-wave research made clear that children could be resilient in one context but not another, at one time but not another, and adaptive in some aspects of their lives and maladaptive in other aspects. Building on first-wave literature, second-wave researchers re-conceptualized resilience as more of a continuum of protective and risk factors across multiple domains (e.g., psychological, physical, interpersonal) rather than discrete traits possessed by certain individuals.

Wave three: Interventions

Whereas first-wave resiliency researchers identified factors associated with resilience and second-wave researchers uncovered the influence of developmental processes and systems on resilience, third-wave researchers focused on interventions and methods of fostering resilience (13). Initially, scholars focused on developing comprehensive theory driven interventions, and later used randomized control or comparison groups to test their theories (21, 22). In general, third-wave resiliency research has been characterized by complex studies exploring the effects of targeted interventions over time.

One important finding of this work is the understanding that key windows of opportunity exist for changing the course of a child's development. For example, researchers found that targeting interventions to elementary school students reduced their antisocial behavior and increased their grades as high school students (23). In addition to identifying windows of opportunity, third-wave researchers also assessed the effectiveness of particular interventions.

In an iconic study employing random assignment with families going through divorce, Sandler et al. (24) showed a manualized program for mothers was associated with higher self-esteem, lower substance use, and greater academic achievement of the children six years post intervention (24). The aforementioned studies are two examples of the increased sophistication of third-wave resiliency research and inform current research. Today, third-wave researchers continue to focus on culturally relevant, deliberately timed, comprehensive interventions intended to foster resilience and promote wellbeing.

Wave four: Gene-environment interactions

The fourth wave of resiliency research is grounded by the theory of probabilistic epigenesis – the idea that development is a bidirectional process occurring across multiple levels of functioning with gene-environment interaction playing a central role (25). In general, fourth-wave resiliency researchers focus on the relationships between pathways to resilience and genes, gene expression, and brain structure, and use statistical modeling to investigate interactions in complex systems (26, 27). This wave is also characterized by interdisciplinary resilience research (e.g., ecology, public health, and emergency services) seeking to respond to national concerns (e.g., terrorism, natural disasters, flu pandemics) (28).

Although still in its early stages, fourth wave research has already yielded information regarding specific gene-environment interactions promoting resilience (29), the neuroscience of stress responsivity (30), and effective ways for preparing societies for major disasters (31). Building on past waves of research, this newest focus of resiliency research will likely transform the understanding and application of resilience science.

DYNAMIC PROCESS

Most modern theorists agree that there is little support for the notion that resilience is exclusively an intrinsic trait and emphasize that resilience is part of a dynamic process (4, 14, 32). Individual models are criticized for justifying the practice of "blaming the victim" who exhibits maladaptive responses without adequately accounting for contextual influences and evidence suggesting those experiencing greater systemic oppression are more are susceptible to experiencing traumatic stress (33-35). A number of authors have pointed to the importance of acknowledging the impact of systemic oppressions on resilience (36-38) and adopting a framework for resilience that is contextually situated (39-41). This evidence also points to the need for further research examining culturally-based protective processes (42) and the ways different cultural dimensions (such as individualism, collectivism, and familism) may mediate resilience in difference ways with different cultural groups (43, 44).

According to Wright and Masten (9) in a dynamic, systems model of development, resilience is understood in context of the continual interactions of the systems within the individual, between the individual and environment, as well as amongst other people and other systems (e.g., educational systems; family resources) (9). The authors suggest that in light of the simultaneous interactions among numerous connected systems, resilience may be best understood as a phenomenon involving a number of processes with the capacity for resilience being distributed across a number of interacting systems (see Table 1). Similarly, Masten10 suggests resiliency is influenced by dynamically interacting systems within the individual and their relationships and connections to other systems, family, community, and culture.

This systems based approach highlights how any number of biological, psychological, or sociocultural factors (i.e., within the individual, family, community, and larger culture) are simultaneously interacting to facilitate one's resilience. That is, how resilient a child is after a motor vehicle accident is determined by the unique interactions between the individual's past and present sociocultural context (e.g., number of resources in their country, exposure to collective trauma, family dynamics) and biological and psychological constructs. A shift in any number of these factors can influence whether an individual responds adaptively in one situation but not the next. Individuals can also be more resilient when confronted with certain kinds of stressors relative to others (e.g., a car accident versus the loss of a loved one) as well as vary in their responses depending on the type of environments (e.g., school versus at home) (45, 46).

These complexities point to the importance of ecological, transactional approaches to understanding resilience (47-50). Transactional perspectives highlight how processes across multiple inter-connected bio-psycho-sociocultural domains that can change over time, interact in a way that changes in one domain may impact all the other domains at any point in a person's development, which could impact their resilience in that moment or across their lifespan (51). In sum, practitioners are encouraged to consider both the cumulative risk factors as well as individual differences when interacting with patients following a motor vehicle accident.

INTERVENTIONS

In the following sections we present guidelines and suggestions for clinicians working with youth who have been involved in motor vehicle accidents and may be at risk for developing symptoms of PTSD. In general, we advocate for a holistic approach which fosters resilience by maintaining balance between focusing on symptoms and instilling hope by drawing upon the child's strengths and unique resources.

STRENGTH-BASED PERSPECTIVE

Perhaps most importantly, clinicians are advised to approach children and adolescents injured in automobile accidents from a strength-based perspective. A strength-based approach is grounded by the idea that humans have a self-righting tendency and move toward health and wellness under all but the most persistently damaging life circumstances (52). Resilience is at the core of a strength-based approach, anchored by the belief that people bounce back from life's challenges despite what may appear to be overwhelming odds (53, 54). Rather than focus solely on deficits, strength-based clinicians search for assets by helping patients identity resources, solutions, and evidence of prior successes in the midst of adversity. The strength-based approach also considers the influence of culture in patients' lives and empowers them to play active roles in healing and recovery.

One important component of a strength-based approach is the clinician's mindset (55). Although medical professionals are well trained in identifying pathology and symptoms of illness, they typically do not receive as much training in recognizing and honoring the strengths and resilience of their patients. The very way a clinician gathers information holds potential to communicate to the child and family what is of greater interest and importance: pathology or resilience (56). Therefore, clinicians using a strengths-based approach make efforts to refrain from focusing only on symptoms, and include inquiry into patient and family resources, supports, strengths, and past examples of adapting to challenges. Likewise, strengths-based models promote focusing on courage, hope, vision, and being mindful of the lifelong impact clinicians may have on their young patients. Clinicians may also help foster patient resilience by searching for and reinforcing what Brooks calls, "Islands of Competence" – specific areas of strength children have developed in response to life challenges (57). Acknowledging and celebrating these "islands" enhances self-esteem and enables children to cope more successfully with life challenges.

Another critical aspect of a strength-based approach, and contained within a resilience mindset, is a clinical relationship grounded by empathy. Because empathy drives human connection, and connection has been well documented to positively impact health and wellness, the importance of empathy within the clinical relationship cannot be overstated. Connection and empathy have been linked to a number of positive health outcomes, such as having beneficial health effects for the cardiovascular, endocrine, and immune systems, as well as positively affecting survival rates among cancer and stroke survivors (58).

Moreover, connection and empathic physician-patient relationships are associated with lower burnout, greater job satisfaction, and lower levels of stress among clinicians (59-61). Thus, empathy is mutually beneficial and bidirectional.

Simply defined, empathy is the capacity to take the perspective of others and understand the world through their eyes (62). Whereas sympathy can be understood as "feeling sorry for," empathy is understood as "feeling sorry with." It is often misunderstood that one must have experienced a similar event in order to be empathic, however to be empathic is to connect to with a similar feeling within oneself, regardless if one has experienced a similar event. Considering motor vehicle accidents for example, when a child describes her experience of being injured in an accident and feeling scared, the clinician need not have also been injured in an accident as a child.

Rather, the clinician recalls the feeling of being scared and connects her own subjective experience of fear with the child's feeling. Connecting with one's own feeling of being scared facilitates responding to the child in an empathic way. Consider the differences between, "You were very fortunate not to have been more seriously injured" and "That sounds very frightening, I'm glad we're able to help." The former is typical of a sympathetic response while the latter is an example of an empathic response. Clinicians are encouraged to practice empathic responding and be mindful of sympathetic responses, which may have the unintended consequence of hindering the patient-clinician relationship.

Effective communication marked by active listening is another aspect of the strength-based approach. In general, active listening requires one to not just hear what is being said, but to also understand the message and meaning being communicated. With children, this involves understanding and validating what they say while avoiding power struggles by refraining from interrupting or suggesting how they should feel (63). Effective communication also includes clinicians explicitly sharing their understanding of the patient's concerns. Clinicians may hold an empathic understanding, but if it is not communicated the clinician will not be perceived as an empathic physician (64). Furthermore, clinicians are encouraged to remain mindful of making assumptions and remain patient as children share their experiences. A symptom of PTSD is avoidance of reminders of the trauma, and children may be hesitant to talk about the accident. As trust in the clinician builds, however, children may feel relief by sharing their memories and releasing some of their pain. It is also important to note that focusing on data-driven processing (e.g., discussing the factual aspects of the situation) rather than focusing on the meaning of the situation is associated with development of PTSD symptoms three months post-accident (65). Therefore, clinicians are strongly encouraged to include questions and discussion about the meaning of the accident in addition to inquiry focused on gathering factual information.

A final tenant of the strength-based approach that is complimentary to all other components, is the intentional focus on instilling hope in patients. Hope is a cornerstone of resilience, a key ingredient in successful recovery from trauma, and what fuels motivation and focus through difficult situations (56). Feelings of hopelessness, by contrast, are associated with negative psychological outcomes, including depression and suicide (66). The clinician working with children who have been involved in motor vehicle accidents will need to be sensitive and find balance between instilling hope and validating suffering. Again, we stress the importance of empathy in the physician-patient relationship as a vehicle for instilling hope despite delivering potentially difficult diagnoses and prognoses. By being grounded in a strength-based approach, embracing a hopeful mindset, practicing empathy, and listening actively, a clinician will be able to honor a child's strengths without trivializing his pain.

FAMILY AND COMMUNITY INVOLVEMENT

One of the strongest and most consistent predictors of resilience in children is the presence of a stable and supportive caregiver (67). Therefore, clinicians treating children who have been injured in motor vehicle accidents are strongly encouraged to enlist the support and resources of available family members to accompany the child on her journey of healing. The family provides a natural shelter, a safe place to express pain, and a support system extending beyond the walls of the clinic. Moreover, the family often functions as a "home base," where setbacks are absorbed, challenges are met, and successes are celebrated. In cases where other family members have also been injured, the healing journey becomes even more meaningful as the accident and subsequent events become part of the collective family memory and family story (56).

Medical providers can harness the power of the family in several ways. First, clinicians are encouraged to directly communicate to the family the important role they play in their child's recovery. While for some families this will be obvious, others may need the encouragement and endorsement from the clinic, and all will benefit from the explicit acknowledgement and reminder of the healing benefit they can provide to their children. For example, clinicians can encourage families to make note of their child's challenges and successes in order to facilitate greater involvement and alleviate some of the isolation the recovering child might feel. Similarly, encouraging families to intentionally make time for talking about the accident and recovery process can help reduce stigma and normalize the process of healing from injury (68). Finally on a systemic level, the clinic might consider hosting annual reunions, or other such events that bring families together to celebrate progress and share their healing journey with other families impacted by motor vehicle accidents and other traumas affecting children.

Supplementing family involvement, clinicians working with youth injured in automobile accidents are advised to encourage patients to reengage with their respective communities as soon as possible. Community involvement becomes all the more important in cases with children who may have lost their family or are without strong familial support. Community, understood as an extension of the family, helps support, guide, and encourage children as they recover from injury and heal from trauma (68). For children, one important area of community involvement occurs through school systems and quick reestablishment of schooling has been endorsed as best-practice for helping children recover from trauma (69, 70).

Clinicians are thus advised to talk with families about returning their children to school as soon as possible and to promptly assist with necessary documentation should the child only be able to return to school on a limited basis. In addition to returning to school, children and families belonging to spiritual and religious communities should be encouraged to reconnect and involve themselves, as much as possible, with their faith community. In general, reengagement with community serves to reestablish pre-trauma routines and normalizes life after trauma, facilitating the healing process (68).

GENDER AND AGE DIFFERENCES

Two final variables for clinicians to consider when working with children injured in motor vehicle accidents are the age and gender of the patient. Although a child's response to trauma is often predicted by the severity of the exposure, sometimes referred to as a "dose-response gradient," it is also influenced by the child's gender and age (56). Differences in responding to traumatic events, and to developing symptoms of PTSD, are thus influenced by the child's developmental stage, cognitive abilities, and emotional regulation strategies.

Regarding age, differences in risk and protective factors can be difficult to interpret and need to be examined on a case-by-case basis. On one hand, young children are often understood to be more physically and psychologically vulnerable than adolescents due to their developmental stage and dependence on caregivers; on the other hand, young children are somewhat protected from trauma by their potentially limited understanding of the event as it unfolds, especially when the family unit remains relatively stable (71).

Conversely, although adolescents are more physically developed compared to younger children, their greater awareness of trauma as it unfolds and what it may mean for their future places them at risk for developing PTSD symptoms (68). However, compared to younger children, adolescents tend to have more sophisticated problem-solving skills, a larger repertoire of emotion regulation strategies, and a larger social support network, all of which are considered protective factors against developing PTSD symptoms (68).

Although research examining gender differences in responding to trauma and developing PTSD symptoms has yielded clearer results, clinicians are nonetheless encouraged to consider patients on a case-by-case basis and remain mindful of cultural influences on the reporting of psychological symptoms. Overall, a large body of literature reveals that women and girls report more psychological symptoms in response to trauma and are approximately twice as likely to meet criteria for a PTSD diagnosis compared to men and boys (72).

This is consistent with epidemiological research revealing higher prevalence of anxiety-based disorders among women in general, including among female adolescents and children compared to men and boys (73-75). Complicating these seemingly straightforward results however, is research indicating that men are less likely than women to report symptoms of and seek help for psychological distress (76). Moreover, men and boys are more likely than women and girls to express posttraumatic distress in the form of anger, irritability, or violent behavior (72). Therefore, clinicians are encouraged to consider how gender and age differences affect a child's understanding and reporting of potential PTSD symptoms following motor vehicle accidents.

CONCLUSION

This review has reviewed the concept of resilience, focusing on how resilience may be understood when working with children and adolescents who have been involved in motor vehicle accidents. Key concepts and terms were defined, including an explanation of risk and protective factors contributing to or hindering resilience. A brief summary of resilience research was provided, tracing the four waves of resilience research through their respective foci on individual characteristics, processes, interventions, and gene-environment interactions. A framework of interventions was suggested grounded by a strength-based perspective incorporating clinical mindset, empathy, active listening, and the intentional focus on installing hope in young patients. Finally, the importance of family and community involvement and consideration of gender and age differences was discussed.

Although over 400,000 children and adolescents are injured yearly in motor vehicle accidents (1) and estimates suggest that between 14-40% of them will develop symptoms of PTSD (77), the majority of these injured youth do not meet diagnostic criteria for PTSD. Furthermore, research indicates psychological factors, rather than injury severity, better predict eventual development and diagnosis of PTSD (3). Thus, clinicians are strongly encouraged to widen their view and look beyond the physical impact of motor vehicle accidents on young people and more fully consider psychological aspects, including strengths, coping strategies, and social supports.

REFERENCES

[1] Safe Kids Worldwide. Motor vehicle safety fact sheet. Washington DC: Children's National Health System, 2016:6.
[2] Keppel-Benson JM, Ollendick TH, Benson MJ. Post-traumatic stress in children following motor vehicle accidents. J Child Psychol Psychiatry 2002;43(2):203-12.
[3] de Vries APJ, Kassam-Adams N, Cnaan A, Sherman-Slate E, Gallagher PR, Winston FK. Looking beyond the physical injury: Posttraumatic stress disorder in children and parents after pediatric traffic injury. Pediatrics 1999;104(6):1293-9.
[4] Masten AS. Ordinary magic: Resilience in development. New York: Guilford, 2014.
[5] Evans GW, Li D, Whipple SS. Cumulative risk and child development. Psychol Bull 2013; 139(6):1342-96.
[6] Obradovic J. How can the study of physiological reactivity contribute to our understanding of adversity and resilience processes in development? Dev Psychopathol 2012;24(02):371-5.

[7] Masten AS, Narayan AJ. Child development in the context of disaster, war, and terrorism: Pathways of risk and resilience. Annu Rev Psychol 2012;63:227-57.
[8] Pine DS, Costello J, Masten A. Trauma, proximity, and developmental psychopathology: the effects of war and terrorism on children. Neuropsychopharmacology 2005;30(10):1781-92.
[9] Wright MO, Masten AS. Pathways to resilience in context. In: Theron LC, Liebenberg L, Ungar M, eds. Youth resilience and culture. Dordrecht: Springer, 2015:3-22.
[10] Masten AS. Ordinary magic: Resilience processes in development. Am Psychol 2001;56(3):227-38.
[11] Masten AS. Global perspectives on resilience in children and youth. Child Dev 2014;85(1):6-20.
[12] Prince-Embury S, Saklofske DH. Resilience in children, adolescents, and adults: Translating research into practice. New York: Springer, 2013.
[13] Wright MO, Masten AS, Narayan AJ. Resilience processes in development: Four waves of research on positive adaptation in the context of adversity. In: Goldstein S, Brooks RB, eds. Handbook of resilience in children. New York: Springer, 2013: 15-37.
[14] Masten AS. Risk and resilience in development. In: Zelazo PD, ed. The Oxford handbook of developmental psychology. NewYork: Oxford University Press, 2014:579-607.
[15] Anthony EJ. The syndrome of the psychologically invulnerable child. In: Anthony EJ, Koupernik C, eds. The child and his family: Children at psychological risk. New York: Wiley, 1974:529-44.
[16] Pines M. In praise of "invulnerables". APA Monitor 1975 Dec:7.
[17] Egeland B, Carlson E, Sroufe LA. Resilience as process. Dev Psychopathol 1993;5(4):517-28.
[18] Masten AS. Resilience comes of age: Reflections on the past and outlook for the next generation of research. In: Glantz MD, Johnson J, Huffman L, eds. Resilience and development: Positive life adaptations. New York: Plenum, 1999:289-96.
[19] Boyce WT, Frank E, Jensen PS, Kessler RC, Nelson CA, Steinberg L, et al. Social context in developmental psychopathology: Recommendations for future research from the Mac Arthur network on psychopathology and development. Dev Psychopathol 1998;10(2):143-64.
[20] Cicchetti D, Rogosch FA. The role of self-organization in the promotion of resilience in maltreated children. Dev Psychopathol 1997;9(4):797-815.
[21] Coie JD, Watt NF, West SG, Hawkins, JD, Asarnow JR, Markman HJ, et al. The science of prevention: A conceptual framework and some directions for a national research program. Am Psychol 1993;48(10):1013-22.
[22] Weissberg RP, Kumpfer KL. Special issue: Prevention that works for children and youth. Am Psychol 2003;58(6-7):425-90.
[23] Hawkins JD, Catalano RF, Kosterman R, Abbott RD, Hill KG. Preventing adolescent health-risk behavior by strengthening protection during childhood. Arch Pediatr Adolesc Med 1999;153(3):226-34.

[24] Sandler I, Wolchik S, Davis C, Haine R, Ayers T. Correlational and experimental study of resilience in children of divorce and parentally bereaved children. In Luthar SS, editor. Resilience and vulnerability: Adaptation in the context of childhood adversities. New York: Cambridge University Press; 2003:213-40.
[25] Gottlieb G. Probabilistic epigenetics. Dev Sci 2007;10(1):1-11.
[26] Charney D. Psychobiological mechanisms of resilience and vulnerability: Implications for successful adaptation to extreme stress. Am J Psychiatry 2004;161(2):195-216.
[27] Feder A, Nestler EJ, Charney DS. Psychobiology and molecular genetics of resilience. Nat Rev Nerurosci 2009;10(6):446-57.
[28] Norris FH, Steven SP, Pfefferbaum B, Wyche KF, Pfefferbaum RL. Community resilience as a metaphor, theory, set of capacities, and strategy for disaster readiness. Am J Commun Psychol 2008;41(1-2):127-50.
[29] Kim-Cohen J, Gold AL. Measured gene-environment interactions and mechanisms promoting resilient development. Curr Dir Psychol Sci 2009;18(3):138-42.
[30] Del Giudice M, Ellis BJ, Shirtcliff EA. The adaptation calibration model of stress responsivity. Neurosci Biobehav Rev 2011;35(7):1562-92.
[31] Masten AS, Obradovic J. Disaster preparation and recovery: Lessons from research on resilience in human development. Ecol Soc 2008;13(1):9.
[32] Panter-Brick C, Leckman JF. Editorial commentary: resilience in child development–interconnected pathways to wellbeing. J Child Psychol Psychiatry 2013;54(4):333-6.
[33] Carter RT. Racism and psychological and emotional injury recognizing and assessing race-based traumatic stress. Couns Psychol 2007;35(1):13-05.
[34] Paradies Y. A systematic review of empirical research on self-reported racism and health. Int J Epidemiol 2006;35(4):888-901.
[35] Utsey SO. Assessing the stressful effects of racism: A review of instrumentation. J Black Psychol 1998;24(3):269-88.
[36] Bockting WO, Miner MH, Swinburne Romine RE, Hamilton A, Coleman E. Stigma, mental health, and resilience in an online sample of the US transgender population. Am J Public Health. 2013;103(5):943-51.
[37] Bowleg L, Huang J, Brooks K, Black A, Burkholder G. Triple jeopardy and beyond: Multiple minority stress and resilience among Black lesbians. J Lesbian Stud 2003;7(4):87-108.
[38] Meyer IH. Identity, stress, and resilience in lesbians, gay men, and bisexuals of color. Couns Psychol 2010;38(3):442-54.
[39] Aponte HJ. Bread & spirit: Therapy with the new poor: Diversity of race, culture, and values. New York: WW Norton, 1994.
[40] Boyd-Franklin N, Bry BH. Reaching out in family therapy: Home-based, school, and community interventions. New York: Guilford, 2012.
[41] Hill RB. The strengths of African American families: Twenty-five years later. Lanham, MD: University Press America, 1999.
[42] Luthar SS. Resilience in development: A synthesis of research across five decades. In: Cicchetti D, Cohen DJ, eds. Developmental psychopathology: Risk, disorder, and adaptation, 2nd ed. Hoboken, NJ: Wiley, 2006:739–95.

[43] Gaines Jr SO, Marelich WD, Bledsoe KL, Steers WN, Henderson MC, Granrose CS, et al. Links between race/ethnicity and cultural values as mediated by racial/ethnic identity and moderated by gender. J Pers Soc Psychol 1997;72(6):1460-76.
[44] Kim UE, Triandis HC, Kâgitçibasi ÇE, Choi SC, Yoon GE. Individualism and collectivism: Theory, method, and applications. Nwbury Park, CA: Sage, 1994.
[45] Luthar SS, Cicchetti D, Becker B. The construct of resilience: A critical evaluation and guidelines for future work. Child Dev 2000;71(3):543-62.
[46] Rutter M. Resilience, competence, and coping. Child Abuse Negl 2007;31(3):205-9.
[47] Cicchetti D. Annual research review: Resilient functioning in maltreated children–past, present, and future perspectives. J Child Psychol Psychiatry 2013;54(4):402-22.
[48] Cowen EL, Durlak JA. Social policy and prevention in mental health. Dev Psychopathol. 2000;12(04):815-34.
[49] Ungar M. Social ecologies and their contribution to resilience. In The social ecology of resilience. New York: Springer, 2012:13-31.
[50] Ungar M, Liebenberg L, Dudding P, Armstrong M, Van de Vijver FJ. Patterns of service use, individual and contextual risk factors, and resilience among adolescents using multiple psychosocial services. Child Abuse Negl 2013;37(2):150-9.
[51] Masten AS, Cicchetti D. Developmental cascades. Dev Psychopathol 2010;22(03):491-5.
[52] Werner EE, Smith RS. Overcoming the odds: High risk children from birth to adulthood. New York: McGraw-Hill, 1992.
[53] Katz M. On playing a poor hand well. New York: Norton, 1997.
[54] Kozol J. Amazing grace: The lives of children and the conscience of a nation. New York: Harper Collins, 1998.
[55] Brooks R. Power of mind-sets: A personal journey to nurture dignity, hope, and resilience in children. In: Crenshaw DA, ed. Reverence in healing: Honoring strengths without trivializing suffering. Lanham, MD: Jason Aronson Rowman Littlefield, 2010:19-40.
[56] Crenshaw DA. A resilience framework for treating severe child trauma. In: Goldstein S, Brooks RB, eds. Handbook of resilience in children. New York: Springer, 2013:309-27.
[57] Brooks R. Children at risk: Fostering resilience and hope. Am J Orthopsychiatry 1994;64(4):545-53.
[58] Uchino BN, Cacioppo JT, Kiecolt-Glaser JK. The relationship between social support systems and physiological processes: A review with emphasis on underlying mechanisms and implications for health. Psychol Bull 1996;119(3):488-531.
[59] Miller MN, McGowen KR. The painful truth: Physicians are not invincible. South Med J 2000; 91(10):966-72.
[60] Zuger A. Dissatisfaction with medical practice. N Engl J Med 2004;350(1):69-75.
[61] Hyyppa MT, Kronholm E, Mattlar C. Mental well-being of good sleepers in a random sample population. Br J Med Psychol 1991;64(1):25-34.
[62] Goleman D. Emotional intelligence: Why it can matter more than IQ. New York: Bantam, 1995.
[63] Goldstein S, Brooks R, DeVries M. Translating resilience theory for application with children and adolescents by parents, teachers, and mental health professionals. In:

Prince-Embury S, Saklofske DH, eds. Resilience in children, adolescents, and adults: Translating research into practice. New York: Springer, 2013:73-90.
[64] Bylund CL, Makoul G. Examining empathy in medical encounters: An observational study using the empathic communication coding system. Health Commun 2005;18(2):123-40.
[65] Ehlers A, Mayou RA, Bryant B. Cognitive predictors of posttraumatic stress disorder in children: Results of a prospective longitudinal study. Behav Res Ther 2003;41(1):1-10.
[66] Hawton K, Casañas i Comabella C, Haw C, Saunders K. Risk factors for suicide in individuals with depression: A systematic review. J Affect Disord 2013;47(1-3):17-28.
[67] Houshyar S, Kaufman J. Resiliency in maltreated children. In: Goldstein S, Brooks RB, eds. Handbook of resilience in children. New York: Springer, 2013:181-200.
[68] Masten AS, Osofsky JD. Disasters and their impact on child development: Introduction to the special section. Child Dev 2010;81(4):1029-39.
[69] Ager A, Stark L, Akesson B, Boothby N. Defining best practices in care and protection of children in crisis-affected settings: A Delphi study. Child Dev 2010;81(4):1271-86.
[70] Kronenberg ME, Hansel TC, Brennan AM, Lawarson B, Osofsky JD. Children of Katrina: Lessons learned about post-disaster symptoms and recovery patterns. Child Dev 2010;81:1241-59.
[71] Osofsky J. Young children and trauma: Interventions and treatment. New York: Guilford, 2004.
[72] Tolin DF, Foa EB. Sex differences in trauma and posttraumatic stress disorder: A quantitative review of 25 years of research. Psychol Bull 2006;132(6):959-92.
[73] Bourdon KH, Boyd JH, Rae DS, Burns BJ, Thompson JW, Locke BZ. Gender differences in phobias: Results of the ECA Community Survey. J Anxiety Disord 1998;2(3):227-41.
[74] Anderson JC, Williams S, McGee R, Silva PA. DSM-III disorders in preadolescent children. Prevalence in a large sample from the general population. Arch Gen Psychiatry 1987;44(1):69-76.
[75] Mcgee R, Feehan M, Williams S, Partridge F, Silva PA, Kelly J. DSM-III disorders in a large sample of adolescents. J Am Acad Child Adolesc Psychiatry 1990;29(4):611-19.
[76] Möller-Leimkühler AM. Barriers to help-seeking by men: a review of sociocultural and clinical literature with particular reference to depression. J Affect Disord 2002;71(1-3):1-9.
[77] Keppel-Benson JM, Ollendick TH, Benson MJ. Post-traumatic stress in children following motor vehicle accidents. J Child Psychol Psychiatry 2002;43(2);203-12.

In: Children and Youth
Editors: Donald E. Greydanus et al.
ISBN: 978-1-53611-102-6
© 2017 Nova Science Publishers, Inc.

Chapter 10

POST-TRAUMATIC STRESS DISORDER AND MOTOR VEHICLE CRASHES IN CHILDREN AND ADOLESCENTS: WHAT DOES THE FUTURE HOLD?

Donald E Greydanus[1],, MD, DrHC(Athens) and Joav Merrick[2-6], MD, MMedSci, DMSc*

[1]Department of Pediatric and Adolescent Medicine,
Western Michigan University Homer Stryker MD School of Medicine,
Kalamazoo, Michigan, US
[2]National Institute of Child Health and Human Development,
Jerusalem, Israel
[3]Health Services, Division for Intellectual and Developmental Disabilities,
Ministry of Social Affairs and Social Services, Jerusalem, Israel
[4]Department of Pediatrics, Mt Scopus Campus,
Hadassah Hebrew University Medical Center, Jerusalem, Israel
[5]Kentucky Children's Hospital, University of Kentucky,
Lexington, Kentucky, US
[6]Center for Healthy Development, School of Public Health,
Georgia State University, Atlanta, US

---

* Correspondence: Donald E. Greydanus, MD, DrHC(Athens), Department of Pediatric and Adolescent Medicine, Western Michigan University Homer Stryker MD School of Medicine, Kalamazoo, MI 49008-1284, United States. E-mail: Donald.greydanus@med.wmich.edu.

The motor vehicle crash is the main cause of death and destruction in children and adolescents. One of the major psychological consequences to those who survive a motor vehicle crash (MVC) is post-traumatic stress disorder (PTSD). This discussion considers the future of research in this field that may also involve the use of artificial intelligence in control of motor vehicles that will take human error out of motor vehicle operation. It is important to consider all means in lowering the death and destruction faced by our children and adolescents on the killing fields of the roads in the United States and the world.

INTRODUCTION

The first steam-powered vehicle is attributed to Ferdinand Verbiest in China and it was made in 1672 for the Kangxi Emperor. The first recorded automobile death was Mary Ward in Ireland who was thrown from a steam-powered car and fell under its wheels in 1869 (1). The first person killed in the United States is recorded as Henry Bliss in New York City on Wednesday, September 13, 1899. The automobile became popular among humans in the 20th century and the motor vehicle crash became the major cause of death and disability among children and adolescents. Research initially focused on the physical trauma that motor vehicle crashes induced, but eventually the psychological toll of MVCs in the pediatric population became appreciated (2). This treatise reflects on how this occurred taking the entire 20th century to be acknowledged by researchers, clinicians, parents, and the general society.

This discussion has continued into the 21st century with more research being accomplished now and into the future of this second decade of this century. Some concepts now being studied will continue to be under researchers' eyes into the near and far future. One issue that continues to be studied is the precise prevalence of PTSD in children and adolescents after motor vehicle crashes. Current data suggest that though the majority of adolescents are exposed to potentially traumatic experiences, most do not develop PTSD (3). However, this "minority" of persons suffering from PTSD remains serious and alarming. Current data suggest that 12% to 46% of school-aged children develop PTSD in the first four months after an MVC and 13% to 25% can also be diagnosed with this condition 4 to 12 months after the MVC (4).

> Real generosity towards the future lies in giving all to the present.
> Albert Camus (1913-1960), Notebooks 1935-1942

WHAT DOES THE FUTURE HOLD?

Precise prevalence rates will continue to be debated by different researchers depending on definitions and methodology that is used. Complicating the prevalence picture is that some develop delayed PTSD beyond the classic development of this condition 1 to 6 months post-trauma (5). Thus, research will further delineate delayed-onset PTSD in contrast to that developing within 6 months. This also highlights the need for improved research with improved scientific study designs to better understand the many complex facets of PTSD and MVCs that complicate the lives of our children (6).

Current work is also focusing on 20th century studies seeking to better understand predictors of PTSD in those who do develop this condition 1 to 6 months post MVC and why others involved in MVCs apparently did not develop it. For example the role of parental psychopathology in the development of childhood PTSD is under review as noted in a recent report that maternal PTSD predicted the presence of the exposed child's PTSD within a month of the accident (7). This remains a complex issue with many variables including whether or not the parent was involved in the MVC, witnessed it, or was not involved in the crash. More understanding on PTSD in children will come from more research into the peri-trauma period of the injury to understand peri-traumatic distress (including peri-traumatic guilt) and its influence on PTSD (8-10).

Another aspect of current and future research is the role of quality of life issues in PTSD development and chronicity. Children with a high degree of body pain and low quality of life (seen on physical and psychosocial scores) tend to have lower health status one year after the MVC (11). The presence of severe pain and/or comorbid psychiatric disorders even with relatively minor physical injury can lead to long-term disability in adults that include PTSD (12, 13). Thus, the need to control pain effectively is an important component in the overall approach to victims of MVCs. The concern for the present and the future is to effectively treat pain related to MVCs without the development of drug addiction in this person (14).

Research tools also need to better identify who needs screening for PTSD since many victims of MVCs continue not be screened for PTSD (15, 16). Early life stress can program the brain to react in heightened ways to stress leading to PTSD and the finding of low cortisol levels in adults with PTSD may reflect earlier trauma in life (17). Research on MVC-induced changes in the HPA axis reflect an initial increase in cortisol followed eventually by a reduction in cortisol levels (17). Current data suggest that a high evening salivary cortisol level with high morning serum interleukin 6 concentrations in children or adolescents involved in a MVC was predictive of PTSD 6 months later (17). Future research will further elicit the neuroendocrine changes seen in persons involved in MVCs that will also be useful in predicting those at risk for psychological complications such as PTSD.

Future studies will continue to assess the role of overt traumatic brain injury (TBI) in the development of changes in the brain and potential influence on psychological effects of MVCs such as PTSD. The link between head injury, loss of consciousness, and PTSD post-MVC will be further explored as current research suggests a positive correlation (18).

Current brain imaging studies (magnetic resonance imaging, diffusional tensor imaging) note changes in white matter thickness and integrity in TBI and these alternations in the central nervous system can have significant effects on the brain and the MVC victim that future studies will clarify (19-22). Future studies will delineate potential PTSD-protective effects of brain-derived neurotrophic factor (protein that is found in the neurotrophic group of growth factors) (23). Also of interest is the findings of neural changes in the anterior cingulate cortex (ACC) of those with PTSD; the ACC is a cerebral structure involved in mechanisms of fear-conditioning (23).

PTSD TREATMENT ISSUES

The management of PTSD in children and adolescents exposed to MVCs remains complex and difficult—requiring more research now and in the future.

Management in the future will be improved by research identifying subgroups of those developing post-trauma symptoms and what treatment works best for each subtype of PTSD (23).The role of parents, teachers, and school psychologists in this process remains under study (24). In addition to pain control, the presence and management of post MVC sleep problems is an important aspect of PTSD management for current and future studies (25).

Efforts to lower the presence of PTSD chronicity need to establish methods to prevent secondary potentially traumatic experiences and improve methods of secondary preventative procedures even in young children (3, 26). The emphasis now and in future studies is and will be to screen and follow MVC persons early; this includes when injury places them in the hospital such as the pediatric intensive care unit (26, 27). The role of anxiety sensitivity in PTSD pathophysiology will continue to be probed (28).

A variety of psychological therapies are used in treating children and adolescents exposed to trauma (i.e., MVCs, sexual assault, civil violence, natural disaster, or family violence). Cognitive-behavioral therapy (CBT) has the best results in research studies but there is no evidence for its effectiveness over a month of treatment—ie, no evidence for long-term efficacy of this or other psychological therapies (29-31). Other psychological therapies that will be further assessed include EMDR (eye movement desensitization and reprocessing), supportive counseling, exposure-based therapy, narrative therapy, debriefing, and psychodynamic therapy (29-32). The use of a diary interventions have been useful in helping with PTSD in post-ICU patients and perhaps can be applied to post-MVC persons as well (33).

Future studies will better identify what kinds of trauma precedes PTSD and what influence single event or repeated trauma has on children and adolescents (29, 30). Consistent and verifiable diagnostic criteria must be used in PTSD diagnosis to help evaluate effective management strategies. The role of psychopharmacologic agents remains under study though the efficacy of these drugs remains quite limited at this time (29, 30, 34-36). Some positive effects in adults have been described in adults with the use of hydrocortisone in PTSD prevention though more research will be conducted in this regard as well as with other medications (34). The role of deep brain stimulation, now being used for various psychiatric disorders, remains to be determined in the future (37).

PTSD PREVENTION IN THE 21ST CENTURY: USE OF ARTIFICIAL INTELLIGENCE

MVCs are the leading cause of death and physical injury in children and adolescents in the United States. This publication has reviewed various aspect of MVCs and PTSD and this chapter considers potential future research development. Efforts to reduce this death and destruction in the killing fields of the American road have been minimal at best. As a well-known group of French (Lyon University) have noted, "a few seconds to have an accident, a long time to recover (38)." Research is underway to make artificial intelligence and self-driving cars a reality in the 21st century (39-42). However, giving up driving will be a great challenge for modern Homo sapiens sapiens! Yet, if society really loves its children and wishes to dramatically reduce this carnage in the 21st century, use of artificial intelligence to control motor vehicles will take the human error out of driving.

> The future depends on what you do today.
> Mahatma Gandhi (1869-1948)

REFERENCES

[1] Setright LJK. Drive on! A social history of the motor car. London: Granta Books, 2004.
[2] Greydanus DE, Merrick J. Post-traumatric stress disorder and motor vehicle accidents. J Pain Manage 2016;9(1):3-10.
[3] McLaughlin KA, Koenen KC, Hill ED, Petukhova M, Sampson NA, Zaslavsky AM, et al. Trauma exposure and posttraumatic stress disorder in a national sample of adolescents. J Am Acad Child Adolesc Psychiatry 2013;52(8):815-30.
[4] Mehta S, Ameratunga SN. Prevalence of post-traumatic stress disorder among children and adolescents who survive road traffic crashes; a systematic review of the international literature. J Paediatr Child Health 2012;48(10):876-85.
[5] Utzon-Frank N, Breinegaard N, Bertelsen M, Borritz M, Eller NH, Nordentoft M, et al. Occurrence of delayed-onset post-traumatic stress disorder: a systematic review and meta-analysis of prospective studies. Scand J Work Environ Health 2014;40(3):215-29.
[6] Scott-Parker B, Senserrick T. A call to improve sampling methodology and reporting in young novice driver research. Inj Pre 2016 Jul 27. pii: injuryprev-2016-042105.
[7] Kolaitis G, Giannakopoulos G, Liakopoulou M, Pervanidou P, Charitaki S, Mihas C, et al. Predicting pediatric posttraumatic stress disorder after road traffic accidents: the role of parental psychopathology. J Trauma Stress 2011;24(4):414-21.
[8] Marsac ML, Kassam-Adams N, Delahanty DL, Widaman KF, Barakat LP. Posttraumatic stress following acute medical trauma in children: A proposed model of bio-psycho-social processes during the peri-trauma period. Clin Child Fam Psychol Rev 2014;17(4):399-411.
[9] Lewis GC, Platts-Mills TF, Liberzon I, Bair E, Swor R, Peak D, et al. Incidence and predictors of acute psychological distress and dissociation after motor vehicle collision: a cross-sectional study. J Trauma Dissociation 2014;15(5):527-47.
[10] Haag AC, Zehnder D, Landolt MA. Guilt is associated with acute stress symptoms in children after road traffic accidents. Eur J Psychotraumatol 2015 Oct 28;6:29074. doi: 10.3402/ejpt.v6.29074.
[11] Batailler P, Hours M, Maza M, Charnay P, Tardy H, Tournier C, et al. Health status recovery at one year in children injured in a road accident: a cohort study. Accid Anal Prev 2014;71:267-72.
[12] Kenardy J, Heron-Delaney M, Warren J, Brown EA. Effect of mental health on long-term disability after a road traffic crash: results from the UQ SuPPORT study. Arch Phys Med Rehabil 2015;96(3):410-7.

[13] Parker AM, Sricharoenchai T, Raparla S, Schneck KW, Bienvenu OJ, Needham DM. Posttraumatic stress disorder in critical illness survivors: A metaanalysis. Crit Care Med 2015;43(5):1121-9.
[14] Roland CL, Setnik B, Brown DA. Assessing the impact of abuse-deterrent opioids (ADOs): identifying epidemiologic factors related to new entrants with low population exposure. Postgrad Med 2016 Dec 14. [Epub ahead of print].
[15] Tierens M, Bal S, Crombez G, Van de Voorde P, Rosseell Y, Antrop I, et al. The traumatic impact of motor vehicle accidents in high school students. J Pediatr Psychol 2012;37(1):1-10.
[16] Odenbach J, Newton A, Gokiert R, Falconer C, Courchesne C, Campbell S, et al. Screening for post-traumatic stress disorder after injury in the pediatric emergency department—a systematic review protocol. Syst Rev 2014;3:19. doi: 10.1186/2046-4053-3-19.
[17] Pervanidoui P, Chrousos GP. Posttraumatic stress disorder in children and adolescents: Neuroendocrine perspectives. Sci Signal 2012;5(245):pt 6. doi: 10.1126/scisignal.2003327.
[18] Roitman P, Gilad M, Ankri YL, Shalev AY. Head injury and loss of consciousness raise the likelihood of developing and maintaining PTSD symptoms. J Trauma Stress 2013;26(6):727-34.
[19] Wang X, Xie H, Cotton AS, Tamburrino MB, Brickman KR, Lewis TJ, et al. Early cortical thickness change after mild traumatic brain injury following motor vehicle collision. J Neurotrauma 2015;32(7):455-63.
[20] Hu H, Zhou Y, Wang Q, Su S, Qiu Y, Ge J, et al. Association of abnormal white matter integrity in the acute phase of motor vehicle accidents with post-traumatic stress disorder. J Affect Disord 2016;190:714-22.
[21] Hruska B, Irish LA, Pacella ML, Sledjeski EM, Delahanty DL. PTSD symptom severity and psychiatric comorbidity in recent motor vehicle accident victims: a latent class analysis. J Anxiety Disord 2014;28(7):644-9.
[22] Boccia M, Piccardi L, Cordellieri P, Guariglia C, Giannini AM. EMDR therapy after motor vehicle accidents: meta-analystic evidence for specific treatment. Front Hum Neurosci 2015 Apr 21:213. doi: 10.3389/fnhum.2015.00213.
[23] Su S, Xiao Z, Lin Z, Qui Y, Jin Y, Wang Z. Plasma-brain derived neurotrophic factor levels in patients suffering from post-traumatic stress disorder. Psychiatry Res 2015;229(1-2):365-9.
[24] Alisic E. Teachers' perspectives on providing support to children after trauma: a qualitative study. Sch Psychol Q 2012;27(1):51-9.
[25] Wittmann L, Zehnder D, Jenni OG, Landolt MA. Predictors of children's sleep onset and maintenance of problems after road traffic accidents. Eur J Psychotraumatol 2012;3. doi: 10.3402/ejpt.v3i0.8402.
[26] Kramer DN, Hertli MB, Landolt MA. Evaluation of an early risk screener for PTSD in preschool children after accidental injury. Pediatrics 2013;132(4):e945-51.
[27] Dow BL, Kenardy JA, Le Brocque RM, Long DA. The utility of Children's Revised Impact of Event Scale in screening for concurrent PTSD following admission to intensive care. J Trauma Stress 2012;25(5):602-5.

[28] Olatunji BO, Fan Q. Anxiety sensitivity and post-traumatic stress reactions: evidence for intrusions and physiologic arousal as mediating and moderating mechanisms. J Anxiety Disord 2015;34:76-85.
[29] Gillies D, Taylor F, Gray C, O'Brien L, D'Abrew N. Psychological therapies for the treatment of post-traumatic stress disorder in children and adolescents. Cochrane Database Syst Rev 2012;12:CD006726. doi: 10.1002/14651858.CD006726.pub2.
[30] Gillies D, Taylor F, Gray C, O'Brien L, D'Abrew N. Psychological therapies for the treatment of post-traumatic stress disorder in children and adolescents. Evid Based Child Health 2013;8(3):1004-116.
[31] Bisson JI, Roberts NP, Andrew M, Lewis C. Psychological therapies for chronic post-traumatic stress disorder (PTSD) in adults. Cochrane Database Syst Rev 2013;12:CD003388. doi: 10.1002/14651858.CD003388.pub.4.
[32] Pfefferbaum B, Jacobs AK, Kitiéma P, Everly GS Jr. Child debriefing: A review of the evidence base. Prehosp Disaster Med 2015;30(3):306-15.
[33] Mehlhorn J, Freytag A, Schmidt K, Brunkhorst FM, Graf J, Troitzsch U, et al. Rehabilitation interventions for postintensive care syndrome: A systematic review. Crit Care Med 2014;42(5):1263-71.
[34] Amos T, Stein DJ, Ipser JC. Pharmacologic interventions for preventing post-traumatic stress disorder (PTSD). Cochrane Database Syst Rev 2014;7:CD006239. doi: 10. 1002/14651858.CD006239.pub2.
[35] Forman-Hoffman V, Knauer S, McKeenan J, Zolotor A, Bianco R, Lloyd S, et al. Child and adolescent exposure to trauma: comparative effectiveness of interventions addressing trauma other than maltreatment or family violence. Rockville, MD: Agency Healthcare Research Quality, Report No: 13-EHC054-EF, 2013.
[36] Kassam-Adams N, Marsac ML, Hildenbrand A, Winston FK. Postraumatic stress following pediatric injury: update on diagnosis, risk factors, and intervention. JAMA Pediatr 2013;167(12):1158-65.
[37] Reznikov R, Hamani C. Posttraumatic stress disorder: perspectives for use of deep brain stimulation. Neuromodulation 2016 Dec 19. doi: 10.1111/ner12551. [Epub ahead of print].
[38] Tournier C, Charnay P, Tardy H, Chossegros L, Carnis L, Hours M. A few seconds to have an accident, a long time to recover: Consequences to road victims from the ESPARR cohort 2 years after the accicent. Accid Anal Prev 2014;72:422-32.
[39] Wagner A, Oftman S, Maxfield R. From the primordial soup to self-driving cares: standards and their role in natural and technological innovation. J R Soc Interface 2016 Feb;13(115):20151086. doi: 10.1098/rsif.2015.1086.
[40] Shladover SE. The truth about "self-driving" cars. Sci Am 2016;314(6):52-7.
[41] Sheridan TB. Human-robot interaction: status and challenges. Hum Factors 2016;58(4):525-32.
[42] Gogolf J, Müller JF. Autonomous cars: in favor of a mandatory ethics-setting. Sci Eng Ethics 2016 July 14. [Epub ahead of print].

SECTION TWO: ACKNOWLEDGMENTS

In: Children and Youth
Editors: Donald E. Greydanus et al.

ISBN: 978-1-53611-102-6
© 2017 Nova Science Publishers, Inc.

Chapter 11

ABOUT THE EDITORS

Donald E. Greydanus, MD, Dr. HC (Athens), FAAP, FSAM (Emeritus), FIAP (HON) is Professor and Founding Chair of the Department of Pediatric and Adolescent Medicine, as well as Pediatrics Program Director at the Western Michigan University Homer Stryker MD School of Medicine (WMED), Kalamazoo, Michigan, USA. He is also Professor of Pediatrics and Human Development at Michigan State University College of Human Medicine (East Lansing, Michigan, USA) as well as Clinical Professor of Pediatrics at MSU College of Osteopathic Medicine in East Lansing, Michigan, USA. Received the 1995 American Academy of Pediatrics' Adele D. Hofmann Award for "Distinquished Contributions in Adolescent Health", the 2000 Mayo Clinic Pediatrics Honored Alumnus Award for "National Contributions to the field of Pediatrics," and the 2003 William B Weil, Jr., MD Endowed Distinguished Pediatric Faculty Award from Michigan State University College of Medicine for "National and international recognition as well as exemplary scholarship in pediatrics." Received the 2004 Charles R Drew School of Medicine (Los Angeles, CA) Stellar Award for contributions to pediatric resident education and awarded an honorary membership in the Indian Academy of Pediatrics—an honor granted to only a few pediatricians outside of India. Was the 2007-2010 Visiting Professor of Pediatrics at Athens University, Athens, Greece and received the Michigan State University College of Human Medicine Outstanding Community Faculty Award in 2008. In 2010 he received the title of Doctor Honoris Causa from the University of Athens (Greece) as a "distinguished scientist who through outstanding work has bestowed praise and credit on the field of adolescent medicine (Ephebiatrics)." In 2010 he received the

Outstanding Achievement in Adolescent Medicine Award from the Society for Adolescent Medicine "as a leading force in the field of adolescent medicine and health." In 2014 he was selected by the American Medical Association as AMA nominee for the ACGME Pediatrics Residency Review Committee (RRC) in Chicago, Illinois, USA. Past Chair of the National Conference and Exhibition Planning Group (Committee on Scientific Meetings) of the American Academy of Pediatrics and member of the Pediatric Academic Societies' (SPR/PAS) Planning Committee (1998 to Present). In 2011 elected to The Alpha Omega Alpha Honor Society (Faculty member) at Michigan State University College of Human Medicine, East Lansing, Michigan. Former member of the Appeals Committee for the Pediatrics' Residency Review Committee (RRC) of the Accreditation Council for Graduate Medical Education (Chicago, IL) in both adolescent medicine and general pediatrics. Numerous publications in adolescent health and lectureships in many countries on adolescent health. Email: donald.greydanus@med.wmich.edu

Roger W Apple, PhD, is an assistant professor, licensed psychologist and director of the Pediatric Psychology program in the Department of Pediatric and Adolescent Medicine at the Western Michigan University Homer Stryker MD School of Medicine (WMED), Kalamazoo, Michigan, United States. He was born and raised in southwest Michigan, attended Western Michigan Univerisity earning his PhD in counseling psychology in 2009. During his training he completed a practicum and was employed at Michigan State Univeristy/ Kalamazoo Center for Medical Studies. His research interests include the physician-patient relationship, psychosocial adaptatin to chronic illness and his dissertation was published in 2009 titled *Adolescents' experience of the factors influencing their diabetes treatment regimen.* He has multiple publications including book chapters, editorials, review articles and has presented at multiple pediatric Grand Rounds and lectures. Email: roger.apple@med.wmich.edu

Kathryn White, MA, is a psychologist who has worked in the Pediatric Pscyhology Department for six years at Western Michigan University Homer Stryker MD School of Medicine (WMED), Kalamazoo, Michigan, United States. She has completed several chapters for a variety of books and publications in the field of pediatrics. She has also worked for fourteen years as a deputy for the Cass County Sheriffs Department, Cassopolis, Michigan, United States. Email: kathryn.white@med.wmich.edu.

Joav Merrick, MD, MMedSci, DMSc, born and educated in Denmark is professor of pediatrics, child health and human development, Division of Pediatrics, Hadassah Hebrew University Medical Center, Mt Scopus Campus, Jerusalem, Israel and Kentucky Children's Hospital, University of Kentucky, Lexington, Kentucky United States and professor of public health at the Center for Healthy Development, School of Public Health, Georgia State University, Atlanta, United States, the medical director of the Health Services, Division for Intellectual and Developmental Disabilities, Ministry of Social Affairs and Social Services, Jerusalem, the founder and director of the National Institute of Child Health and Human Development in Israel. Numerous publications in the field of pediatrics, child health and human development, rehabilitation, intellectual disability, disability, health, welfare, abuse, advocacy, quality of life and prevention. Received the Peter Sabroe Child Award for outstanding work on behalf of Danish Children in 1985 and the International LEGO-Prize ("The Children's Nobel Prize") for an extraordinary contribution towards improvement in child welfare and well-being in 1987. Email: jmerrick@zahav.net.il

In: Children and Youth
Editors: Donald E. Greydanus et al.
ISBN: 978-1-53611-102-6
© 2017 Nova Science Publishers, Inc.

Chapter 12

ABOUT THE DEPARTMENT OF PEDIATRIC AND ADOLESCENT MEDICINE, WESTERN MICHIGAN UNIVERSITY HOMER STRYKER MD SCHOOL OF MEDICINE (WMED), KALAMAZOO, MICHIGAN, UNITED STATES

Mission and service

The Western Michigan University Homer Stryker MD School of Medicine was started in 2012 and its first class of medical students began in 2014. The Department of Pediatric and Adolescent Medicine has a pediatric residency program which is accredited by the Accreditation Council for Graduate Medical Education (ACGME) in Chicago, Illinois, USA and the current residency program in Pediatrics started in 1990.

The WMED Department of Pediatric and Adolescent Medicine has a commitment to a comprehensive approach to the health and development of the child, adolescent, and the family. The Department has a blend of academic general pediatricians and pediatric specialists. Our Pediatric Clinic team provides a broad spectrum of general well and sick child care (birth through 18 years) including immunizations, monitoring general physical and emotional growth, motor skill development, sports medicine (including participation evaluations and evaluation of common sports injuries), child abuse evaluations, and psychosocial or behavioral assessment. WMED Pediatrics believes in immunizations as a protection against preventative disease processes. Our Pediatrics Clinic is undergoing a transformation to a patient-centered medical home (PCMH). A patient-centered medical home is a way to deliver coordinated and comprehensive primary care to our infants, children, adolescents and young adults. It is a partnership between individuals and families within a health care setting, which allows for a more efficient use of resources and time to improve the quality of outcomes for all involved through care provided by a continuity care team.

Research activities

The Department has a variety of research projects in adolescent medicine, neurobehavioral pediatrics, adolescent gynecology, pediatric diabetes mellitus, asthma, and cystic fibrosis. The WMED Department of Pediatric and Adolescent Medicine has published a number of medical textbooks: Essential adolescent medicine (McGraw-Hill Medical Publishers), The pediatric diagnostic examination (McGraw-Hill), Pediatric and adolescent psychopharmacology (Cambridge University Press), Behavioral pediatrics, 2nd edition (iUniverse Publishers in New York and Lincoln, Nebraska), Behavioral pediatrics 3rd edition (New York: Nova Biomedical Books); 4th Edition: In press. Pediatric practice: Sports medicine (McGraw-Hill), Handbook of clinical pediatrics (Singapore: World Scientific), Neurodevelopmental disabilities: Clinical care for children and young adults (Dordrecht: Springer), Adolescent medicine: Pharmacotherapeutics in medical disorders (Berlin/Boston: De Gruyter), Adolescent medicine: Pharmacotherapeutics in general, mental, and sexual health (Berlin/Boston: De Gruyter), Pediatric psychodermatology (Berlin/Boston: De Gruyter), Substance abuse in adolescents and young adults: A manual for pediatric and primary care clinicians (Berlin/Boston: De Gruyter), and tropical pediatrics (New York: Nova); Second edition in press.

    The Department has edited a number of journal issues published by Elsevier Publishers covering pulmonology (State of the Art Reviews: Adolescent Medicine—AM:STARS), genetic disorders in adolescents (AM:STARS), neurologic/neurodevelopmental disorders (AM:STARS), behavioral pediatrics (Pediatric Clinics of North America), pediatric psychopharmacology in the 21st century (Pediatric Clinic of North America), nephrologic disorders in adolescents (AM:STARS), college health (Pediatric Clinics of North America), adolescent medicine (Primary Care: Clinics in Office Practice), behavioral pediatrics in children and adolescents (Primary Care: Clinics in Office Practice), adolescents and sports (Pediatric Clinics of

North America), and developmental disabilities (Pediatric Clinics of North America). The Department has also edited a journal issue on musculoskeletal disorders in children and adolescents for the American Academy of Pediatrics' AM:STARs; in April of 2013 a Subspecialty Update issue was published in AM:STARs.

The department has developed academic ties with a variety of international medical centers and organizations, including the Queen Elizabeth Hospital in Hong Kong, Indian Academy of Pediatrics (New Delhi, India), the University of Athens Children's Hospital (First and Second Departments of Paediatrics) in Athens, Greece and the National Institute of Child Health and Human Development in Jerusalem, Israel.

Contact

Professor Dilip R Patel, MD and professor Donald E Greydanus, MD
Department of Pediatric and Adolescent Medicine
Western Michigan University Homer Stryker MD School of Medicine
1000 Oakland Drive, D48G, Kalamazoo, MI 49008-1284, United States
Email: Donald.greydanus@med.wmich.edu and dilip.Patel@med.wmich.edu
Website: http://www.med.wmich.edu

In: Children and Youth
Editors: Donald E. Greydanus et al.
ISBN: 978-1-53611-102-6
© 2017 Nova Science Publishers, Inc.

Chapter 13

ABOUT THE NATIONAL INSTITUTE OF CHILD HEALTH AND HUMAN DEVELOPMENT IN ISRAEL

The National Institute of Child Health and Human Development (NICHD) in Israel was established in 1998 as a virtual institute under the auspices of the Medical Director, Ministry of Social Affairs and Social Services in order to function as the research arm for the Office of the Medical Director. In 1998 the National Council for Child Health and Pediatrics, Ministry of Health and in 1999 the Director General and Deputy Director General of the Ministry of Health endorsed the establishment of the NICHD.

Mission

The mission of a National Institute for Child Health and Human Development in Israel is to provide an academic focal point for the scholarly interdisciplinary study of child life, health, public health, welfare, disability, rehabilitation, intellectual disability and related aspects of human development. This mission includes research, teaching, clinical work, information and public service activities in the field of child health and human development.

Service and academic activities

Over the years many activities became focused in the south of Israel due to collaboration with various professionals at the Faculty of Health Sciences (FOHS) at the Ben Gurion University of the Negev (BGU). Since 2000 an affiliation with the Zusman Child Development Center at the Pediatric Division of Soroka University Medical Center has resulted in collaboration around the establishment of the Down Syndrome Clinic at that center. In 2002 a full course on "Disability" was established at the Recanati School for Allied Professions in the Community, FOHS, BGU and in 2005 collaboration was started with the Primary Care Unit of the faculty and disability became part of the master of public health course on "Children and society". In the academic year 2005-2006 a one semester course on "Aging with disability" was started as part of the master of science program in gerontology in our collaboration with the Center for Multidisciplinary Research in Aging. In 2010 collaborations with the Division of Pediatrics, Hadassah Hebrew University Medical Center, Jerusalem, Israel around the National Down Syndrome Center and teaching students and residents about intellectual and developmental disabilities as part of their training at this campus.

Research activities

The affiliated staff have over the years published work from projects and research activities in this national and international collaboration. In the year 2000 the International Journal of Adolescent Medicine and Health and in 2005 the International Journal on Disability and Human Development of De Gruyter Publishing House (Berlin and New York) were affiliated with the National Institute of Child Health and Human Development. From 2008 also the International Journal of Child Health and Human Development (Nova Science, New York), the International Journal of Child and Adolescent Health (Nova Science) and the Journal of Pain Management (Nova Science) affiliated and from 2009 the International Public Health Journal (Nova Science) and Journal of Alternative Medicine Research (Nova Science). All peer-reviewed international journals.

National collaborations

Nationally the NICHD works in collaboration with the Faculty of Health Sciences, Ben Gurion University of the Negev; Department of Physical Therapy, Sackler School of Medicine, Tel Aviv University; Autism Center, Assaf HaRofeh Medical Center; National Rett and PKU Centers at Chaim Sheba Medical Center, Tel HaShomer; Department of Physiotherapy, Haifa University; Department of Education, Bar Ilan University, Ramat Gan, Faculty of Social Sciences and Health Sciences; College of Judea and Samaria in Ariel and in 2011 affiliation with Center for Pediatric Chronic Diseases and National Center for Down Syndrome, Department of Pediatrics, Hadassah Hebrew University Medical Center, Mount Scopus Campus, Jerusalem.

International collaborations

Internationally with the Department of Disability and Human Development, College of Applied Health Sciences, University of Illinois at Chicago; Strong Center for Developmental Disabilities, Golisano Children's Hospital at Strong, University of Rochester School of Medicine and Dentistry, New York; Centre on Intellectual Disabilities, University of Albany, New York; Centre for Chronic Disease Prevention and Control, Health Canada, Ottawa; Chandler Medical Center and Children's Hospital, Kentucky Children's Hospital, Section of Adolescent Medicine, University of Kentucky, Lexington; Chronic Disease Prevention and Control Research Center, Baylor College of Medicine, Houston, Texas; Division of Neuroscience, Department of Psychiatry, Columbia University, New York; Institute for the Study of Disadvantage and Disability, Atlanta; Center for Autism and Related Disorders, Department Psychiatry, Children's Hospital Boston, Boston; Department of Pediatric and Adolescent Medicine, Western Michigan University Homer Stryker MD School of Medicine, Kalamazoo, Michigan, United States; Department of Paediatrics, Child Health and Adolescent Medicine, Children's Hospital at Westmead, Westmead, Australia; International Centre for the Study of Occupational and Mental Health, Düsseldorf, Germany; Centre for Advanced Studies in Nursing, Department of General Practice and Primary Care, University of Aberdeen, Aberdeen, United Kingdom; Quality of Life Research Center, Copenhagen, Denmark; Nordic School of Public Health, Gottenburg, Sweden, Scandinavian Institute of Quality of Working Life, Oslo, Norway;

The Department of Applied Social Sciences (APSS) of The Hong Kong Polytechnic University Hong Kong.

Targets

Our focus is on research, international collaborations, clinical work, teaching and policy in health, disability and human development and to establish the NICHD as a permanent institute in Israel in order to conduct model research and together with the four university schools of public health/medicine in Israel establish a national master and doctoral program in disability and human development at the institute to secure the next generation of professionals working in this often non-prestigious/low-status field of work.

Contact

Joav Merrick, MD, MMedSci, DMSc
Professor of Pediatrics
Medical Director, Health Services, Division for Intellectual and Developmental Disabilities, Ministry of Social Affairs and Social Services, POB 1260, IL-91012 Jerusalem, Israel.
E-mail: jmerrick@zahav.net.il

In: Children and Youth
Editors: Donald E. Greydanus et al.
ISBN: 978-1-53611-102-6
© 2017 Nova Science Publishers, Inc.

Chapter 14

ABOUT THE BOOK SERIES "PEDIATRICS, CHILD AND ADOLESCENT HEALTH"

Pediatrics, child and adolescent health is a book series with publications from a multidisciplinary group of researchers, practitioners and clinicians for an international professional forum interested in the broad spectrum of pediatric medicine, child health, adolescent health and human development.

- Merrick J, ed. Child and adolescent health yearbook 2011. New York: Nova Science, 2012.
- Merrick J, ed. Child and adolescent health yearbook 2012. New York: Nova Science, 2012.
- Roach RR, Greydanus DE, Patel DR, Homnick DN, Merrick J, eds. Tropical pediatrics. A public health concern of international proportions. New York: Nova Science, 2012.
- Merrick J, ed. Child health and human development yearbook 2011. New York: Nova Science, 2012.
- Merrick J, ed. Child health and human development yearbook 2012. New York: Nova Science, 2012.
- Shek DTL, Sun RCF, Merrick J, eds. Developmental issues in Chinese adolescents. New York: Nova Science, 2012.
- Shek DTL, Sun RCF, Merrick J, eds. Positive youth development: Theory, research and application. New York: Nova Science, 2012.
- Zachor DA, Merrick J, eds. Understanding autism spectrum disorder: Current research aspects. New York: Nova Science, 2012.
- Ma HK, Shek DTL, Merrick J, eds. Positive youth development: A new school curriculum to tackle adolescent developmental issues. New York: Nova Science, 2012.

- Wood D, Reiss JG, Ferris ME, Edwards LR, Merrick J, eds. Transition from pediatric to adult medical care. New York: Nova Science, 2012.
- Isenberg Y. Guidelines for the healthy integration of the ill child in the educational system: Experience from Israel. New York: Nova Science, 2013.
- Shek DTL, Sun RCF, Merrick J, eds. Chinese adolescent development: Economic disadvantages, parents and intrapersonal development. New York: Nova Science, 2013.
- Shek DTL, Sun RCF, Merrick J, eds. University and college students: Health and development issues for the leaders of tomorrow. New York: Nova Science, 2013.
- Shek DTL, Sun RCF, Merrick J, eds. Adolescence and behavior issues in a Chinese context. New York: Nova Science, 2013.
- Sun J, Buys N, Merrick J. Advances in preterm infant research. New York: Nova Science, 2013.
- Tsitsika A, Janikian M, Greydanus DE, Omar HA, Merrick J, eds. Internet addiction: A public health concern in adolescence. New York: Nova Science, 2013.
- Shek, DTL, Lee TY, Merrick J, eds. Promotion of holistic development of young people in Hong Kong. New York: Nova Science, 2013.
- Shek DTL, Ma C, Lu Y, Merrick J, eds. Human developmental research: Experience from research in Hong Kong. New York: Nova Science, 2013.
- Rubin IL, Merrick J, eds. Child health and human development: Social, economic and environmental factors. New York: Nova Science, 2013.
- Merrick J, ed. Chronic disease and disability in childhood. New York: Nova Science, 2013.
- Rubin IL, Merrick J, eds. Break the cycle of environmental health disparities: Maternal and child health aspects. New York: Nova Science, 2013.
- Rubin IL, Merrick J, eds. Environmental health disparities in children: Asthma, obesity and food. New York: Nova Science, 2013.
- Rubin IL, Merrick J, eds. Environmental health: Home, school and community. New York: Nova Science, 2013.
- Merrick J, Kandel I, Omar HA, eds. Children, violence and bullying: International perspectives. New York: Nova Science, 2013.
- Omar HA, Bowling CH, Merrick J, eds. Playing with fire: Children, adolescents and firesetting. New York: Nova Science, 2013.

About the Book Series "Pediatrics, Child and Adolescent Health"

- Merrick J, Tenenbaum A, Omar HA, eds. School, adolescence and health issues. New York: Nova Science, 2014.
- Merrick J, Tenenbaum A, Omar HA, eds. Adolescence and sexuality: International perspectives. New York: Nova Science, 2014.
- Diamond G, Arbel E. Adoption: The search for a new parenthood adoption. New York: Nova Science, 2014.
- Taylor MF, Pooley JA, Merrick J, eds. Adolescence: Places and spaces. New York: Nova Science, 2014.
- Greydanus DE, Feinberg AN, Merrick J, eds. Born into this world: Health issues. New York: Nova Science, 2014.
- Greydanus DE, Feinberg AN, Merrick J, eds. Caring for the newborn: A comprehensive guide for the clinician. New York: Nova Science, 2014.
- Rubin IL, Merrick J, eds. Environment and hope: Improving health, reducing AIDS and promoting food security in the world. New York: Nova Science, 2014.
- Greydanus DE, Feinberg AN, Merrick J, eds. Pediatric and adolescent dermatology: Some current issues. New York: Nova Science, 2014.
- Roach RR, Greydanus DE, Patel DR, Merrick J, eds. Tropical pediatrics: A public helath concern of international proportions, Second edition. New York: Nova Science, 2015.
- Merrick J, ed. Child and adolescent health issues: A tribute to the pediatrician Donald E Greydanus. New York: Nova Science, 2015.
- Feinberg AN. A pediatric resident pocket guide: Making the most of morning reports. New York: Nova Science, 2015.
- Greydanus DE, Patel DR, Pratt HD, Calles Jr JL, Nazeer A, Merrick J, eds. Behavioral pediatrics, 4th edition. New York: Nova Science, 2015.
- Merrick J, ed. Disability, chronic disease and human development. New York: Nova Science, 2015.
- Hegamin-Younger C, Merrick J, eds. Caribbean adolescents: Some public health concerns. New York: Nova Science, 2015.
- Merrick J, ed. Adolescence and health: Some international perspectives. New York: Nova Science, 2015.
- Omar HA. Youth suicide prevention: Everybody's business. New York: Nova Science, 2015.
- Greydanus DE, Raj VMS, Merrick J, eds. Chronic disease and disability: The pediatric kidney. New York: Nova Science, 2015.
- Merrick J, ed. Children and childhood: Some international aspects. New York: Nova Science, 2016.

- Shek DTL, Lee TY, Merrick J, eds. Children and adolescents: Future challenges. New York: Nova Science, 2016.
- Shek DTL, Wu FKU, Leung JTY, Merrick J, eds. Adolescence: Positive youth development programs in Chinese communities. New York: Nova Science, 2016.
- Merrick J, Greydanus DE, eds. Sexuality: Some international aspects. New York: Nova Science, 2016.
- Harel-Fisch Y, Abdeen Z, Navot M. Growing up in the Middle East: The daily lives and well-being of Israeli and Palestinian youth. New York: Nova Science, 2016.
- Greydanus DE, Malhotra D, Merrick J, eds. Chronic disease and disability: The pediatric heart. New York: Nova Science, 2016.
- Greydanus DE, Kamboj MK, Merrick J, eds. Chronic disease and disability: The pediatric pancreas. New York: Nova Science, 2016.
- Kamboj MK, Greydanus DE, Merrick J, eds. Diabetes mellitus: Childhood and adolescence. New York: Nova Science, 2016.
- Greydanus DE, Palusci VJ, Merrick J, eds. Chronic disease and disability: Abuse and neglect in childhood and adolescence. New York: Nova Science, 2016.
- Greydanus DE, Calles JL Jr, Patel DR, Nazeer A, Merrick J, eds. Clinical aspects of psychopharmacology in childhood and adlescence, second ed. New York: Nova Science, 2016.

Contact

Professor Joav Merrick, MD, MMedSci, DMSc
Medical Director, Medical Services
Division for Intellectual and Developmental Disabilities
Ministry of Social Affairs and Social Services
POBox 1260, IL-91012 Jerusalem, Israel
E-mail: jmerrick@zahav.net.il

Section Three: Index

INDEX

#

20th century, 4, 6, 7, 9, 14, 15, 26, 27, 38, 41, 47, 48, 57, 198, 199
21st century, ix, x, 5, 6, 8, 9, 13, 14, 15, 25, 26, 27, 36, 38, 41, 43, 46, 51, 55, 57, 61, 198, 201, 212

A

abuse, 101, 108, 116, 123, 124, 162, 203, 209, 212
academic learning, 154, 165
academic performance, 160
academic settings, 155, 163
access, 30, 56, 147, 180, 182
accommodations, 155, 159, 160
active listening, 177, 187, 191
acute stress, 10, 11, 18, 19, 21, 87, 92, 112, 113, 129, 132, 157, 174, 202
acute stress disorder, 10, 11, 19, 21, 87, 92, 113, 129, 132, 157, 174
adaptation, 179, 181, 192, 192, 193
ADHD, 42, 44, 59, 67, 69, 113, 158
adjustment, 16, 112, 113, 128, 132, 168
Administration for Children and Families, 116
adolescent development, 30, 55, 219, 220
adolescents, v, x, 3, 4, 5, 7, 9, 11, 12, 13, 14, 15, 16, 17, 19, 20, 21, 22, 25, 29, 30, 33, 38, 39, 49, 52, 54, 57, 58, 59, 60, 64, 65, 68, 71, 72, 73, 75, 77, 78, 80, 81, 82, 83, 84, 85, 86, 87, 88, 91, 92, 96, 103, 105, 108, 110, 114, 115, 116, 117, 119, 120, 121, 122, 126, 129, 131, 132, 135, 136, 142, 145, 148, 150, 151, 153, 154, 155, 171, 174, 177, 178, 181, 186, 190, 191, 192, 194, 195, 198, 200, 201, 202, 203, 204, 212, 219, 220, 221, 222
adulthood, 30, 78, 88, 194
adults, vii, 7, 9, 10, 13, 14, 21, 28, 39, 41, 44, 52, 55, 63, 65, 67, 69, 82, 86, 96, 99, 108, 109, 110, 113, 121, 122, 123, 126, 127, 138, 139, 148, 154, 162, 192, 195, 199, 201, 204, 212
advocacy, 56, 74, 209
affective reactions, 110
age, 5, 8, 26, 27, 28, 30, 32, 33, 37, 38, 39, 40, 47, 50, 51, 52, 53, 54, 55, 56, 58, 62, 63, 65, 70, 71, 73, 74, 77, 78, 80, 81, 82, 83, 84, 93, 99, 101, 102, 103, 108, 111, 114, 121, 125, 136, 137, 138, 143, 146, 150, 153, 154, 157, 189, 190, 191, 192
Age-specific features, 107, 109
aggression, 66, 67, 137
aggressive behavior, 67, 122
alcohol consumption, 37, 47, 73, 82
alcohol use, 35, 37, 61, 71, 73
alertness, 68, 155
alienation, 13

American Psychiatric Association, 7, 11, 16, 18, 89, 96, 98, 99, 105, 116, 132, 150, 174
American Psychological Association (APA), 16, 89, 93, 105, 192
amnesia, 95, 109, 115, 155
amygdala, 12
anger, 8, 13, 42, 43, 67, 95, 102, 104, 109, 111, 141, 162, 190
anterior cingulate cortex, 10, 200
antisocial behavior, 183
anxiety, 7, 8, 9, 10, 11, 13, 87, 91, 92, 93, 104, 108, 111, 112, 113, 117, 123, 128, 131, 136, 137, 140, 141, 142, 143, 144, 147, 158, 172, 190, 200
anxiety disorder, 8, 11, 113, 123
appraisals, 19, 139, 141
arousal, 7, 95, 98, 108, 109, 127, 136, 137, 138, 171, 204
artificial intelligence, x, 198, 201
assault, 14, 108, 201
assessment, x, 10, 19, 58, 91, 100, 101, 105, 109, 111, 116, 117, 121, 128, 135, 140, 141, 160, 161, 172, 174
assets, 174, 179, 181, 186
attention-deficit hyperactivity disorder, 69, 158
attitudes, 33, 34, 67, 74
attribution, 17, 172
autism, 44, 68, 219
Automobile, ix, xi, 4, 15, 44, 46, 55
avoidance, 56, 95, 108, 109, 112, 115, 120, 123, 127, 136, 137, 138, 145, 155, 162, 169, 187
avoidance behavior, 120, 162, 169
awareness, 19, 56, 83, 94, 97, 119, 120, 128, 143, 144, 179, 190

B

BAC, 38, 51, 53
bad habits, 48
behavior therapy, 21, 151
behavioral assessment, 211
behavioral change, 122, 171

behavioral disorders, 152
behavioral manifestations, 171
behaviors, 30, 33, 34, 36, 37, 39, 49, 51, 52, 58, 61, 63, 64, 66, 68, 71, 73, 83, 100, 101, 112, 113, 120, 124, 155, 158, 164, 165, 166, 167, 171, 172
benefits, 13, 54, 146
bias, 60, 69, 128
blame, 95, 126, 129
blood, 5, 27, 38, 43, 51, 66, 73
borderline personality disorder, 42
brain, 10, 12, 17, 67, 86, 123, 148, 165, 184, 199, 200, 203
brain structure, 184
bullying, 220
burnout, 173, 187

C

calibration, 193
campaigns, 36, 52, 85
cancer, 186
cannabis, 6, 30, 32, 37, 38, 39, 40, 41, 42, 51, 52, 55, 65, 66
car accidents, 7, 8, 28
caregivers, 98, 120, 127, 130, 137, 155, 161, 172, 181, 190
causal relationship, 167
CDC, 26, 35, 40, 45, 55, 57, 74, 78, 81, 88, 92, 104, 149
central nervous system, 200
challenges, 108, 109, 112, 115, 164, 179, 186, 188, 189, 204, 222
child abuse, 94, 144, 152, 211
Child Behavior Checklist, 10
child development, 182, 191, 193, 195
child labor, 180
child maltreatment, 142
Child Trauma Screening Questionnaire (CTSQ), 138, 148, 150
childhood, 14, 19, 22, 30, 43, 60, 85, 108, 117, 149, 165, 166, 174, 192, 193, 199, 220, 221, 222
children, v, vi, vii, x, 1, 3, 4, 5, 6, 7, 8, 9, 10, 11, 12, 13, 14, 15, 16, 17, 18, 19, 20, 21,

22, 27, 28, 29, 36, 38, 39, 40, 43, 46, 52, 54, 55, 57, 58, 77, 78, 79, 80, 81, 82, 83, 84, 85, 86, 87, 88, 91, 92, 93, 94, 96, 97, 98, 99, 100, 101, 102, 103, 105, 107, 108, 109, 110, 111, 112, 113, 114, 115, 116, 117, 119, 120, 121, 122, 123, 124, 125, 126,
Children's Revised Impact of Events Scale (CRIES), 10, 138, 148, 151
China, ix, 3, 4, 22, 132, 198
chronic illness, 182, 208
clarity, 122, 159
classroom, vi, 130, 153, 155, 158, 159, 160, 162, 163, 164, 166, 167, 168, 169, 171, 172
Clinical implications, 115
clinical presentation, 108, 111
clusters, 113, 136, 155
cocaine, 38, 52
cognition, 31, 109
cognitive abilities, 181, 182, 190
Cognitive Behavioral Intervention for Trauma in Schools (CBITS), 147
Cognitive behavioral therapy (CBT), 140, 142, 143, 145, 146, 147, 149, 201
cognitive capacities, 166
cognitive development, 166
cognitive function, 126, 179
cognitive impairment, 103
cognitive model of posttraumatic stress disorder, 142, 150
cognitive processing, 144
cognitive profile, 163, 166, 167
cognitive skills, 30, 125
cognitive variables, 19
cognitive-behavioral therapy, 13, 151, 152
collaboration, 155, 161, 172, 173, 216, 217
collectivism, 184, 194
college students, 38, 41, 45, 66, 73, 220
collision-related play, 171
collisions, xi, 15, 46, 55, 67, 70, 81, 85, 154, 155, 158, 159, 160
communication, 52, 67, 145, 165, 187, 195

community, vii, 16, 42, 45, 54, 110, 114, 154, 179, 180, 182, 185, 188, 189, 191, 193, 220, 222
comorbidity, 107, 108, 113, 117, 123, 158, 203
comprehension, 6, 165, 166
conceptual model, 75
conceptualization, 156, 164
concordance, 114
conditioning, 10, 200
conduct disorder, 31, 113
consolidation, 144, 145
control condition, 148
control group, 139, 140, 141, 143, 145, 148
controlled trials, 146
conversations, 64, 95, 127
coping strategies, 142, 178, 191
correlates, 60, 65, 116, 159, 162, 163, 181, 182
cortisol, 12, 19, 199
cost, 6, 9, 16, 27, 30, 57, 138, 140, 146
counseling, 201, 208
counseling psychology, 208
CRF, 103
critical period, 112
cross-sectional study, 18, 202
cues, 94, 97, 114
cultural differences, 60
cultural influence, 190
cultural values, 144, 194
culture, 119, 120, 178, 182, 185, 186, 192, 193

D

danger, 36, 43, 55, 124, 127, 145, 167, 168
death rate, 6, 28, 29, 45
deaths, 5, 6, 15, 25, 26, 27, 28, 29, 30, 31, 32, 33, 36, 38, 39, 44, 45, 50, 52, 53, 55, 57, 58, 70, 74, 82, 154
Debriefing, 139, 142
deep brain stimulation, 201, 204
deficit, 31, 42, 44, 60, 68, 69, 158
Department of Transportation, 39, 41, 48, 57, 58, 59, 65, 173

depersonalization, 102
depression, 7, 8, 10, 13, 34, 69, 102, 104, 113, 128, 130, 131, 141, 142, 143, 147, 158, 162, 188, 195
depressive symptoms, 120
desensitization, 148, 152, 161, 201
destruction, 39, 198, 201
detachment, 95, 109, 136
detection, 73, 88, 107, 109, 110, 111, 116, 152
deterrence, 54, 73
developing brain, 162
developmental process, 183
developmental psychology, 192
developmental psychopathology, 192
diabetes, 43, 68, 208, 212, 222
Diagnostic and Statistical Manual of Mental Disorders, 7, 18, 96, 98, 99, 123, 127
diagnostic criteria, 93, 94, 97, 108, 109, 129, 131, 156, 159, 191, 201
differential diagnosis, 92, 104, 107, 112, 115, 116
direct observation, 162
disability, x, 4, 6, 68, 69, 78, 113, 149, 198, 199, 202, 209, 215, 216, 218, 220, 221, 222
disaster, 113, 117, 150, 192, 193, 195
disorder, v, vi, x, xi, 7, 10, 11, 14, 15, 16, 17, 18, 19, 20, 21, 31, 42, 43, 44, 57, 60, 68, 69, 87, 91, 92, 93, 94, 97, 99, 100, 104, 105, 108, 109, 110, 112, 113, 116, 117, 120, 121, 123, 124, 128, 129, 130, 131, 132, 135, 136, 138, 142, 148, 150, 151, 152, 155, 157, 158, 163, 167, 170, 174, 175, 191, 193, 195, 202, 203, 204, 219
disposition, 178
dissociation, 18, 109, 202
distortions, 142
distress, 10, 96, 98, 102, 109, 120, 123, 125, 127, 129, 133, 137, 140, 149, 155, 160, 161, 162, 169, 179, 190, 199
divergence, 12, 19
domestic violence, 162
DOT, 41, 65, 66

dreaming, 157, 171
drug abuse, 39
drug addiction, 199
drug dependence, 42
drugs, 6, 29, 30, 32, 37, 38, 39, 41, 42, 45, 51, 52, 55, 66, 73, 95, 201
DSM, 7, 16, 94, 97, 99, 119, 121, 126, 127, 128
DSM-IV-TR, 11, 19, 105, 121, 126
dualism, 166, 167
DWI, 31, 32, 51, 53, 65
dysphoria, 109
dysthymic disorder, 113

E

early intervention, vi, 135, 139, 140, 141, 142, 147, 151
education, 36, 42, 44, 47, 48, 49, 50, 54, 55, 70, 71, 123, 145, 180, 207
educational experience, 173
educational settings, 154
educational system, 184, 220
educators, 153, 154, 155, 156, 157, 158, 159, 160, 161, 162, 163, 164, 165, 169, 170, 171, 172, 173, 174
elementary school, 18, 116, 150, 183
emergency, 6, 19, 29, 62, 78, 92, 114, 136, 138, 179, 180, 184, 203
emergency response, 180
emotion regulation, 190
emotional distress, 152
emotional problems, 117, 122
emotional state, 95, 136
empathy, 177, 186, 187, 188, 191, 195
enforcement, 45, 47, 54, 56, 73
environment, 155, 162, 168, 170, 172, 183, 184, 191, 193
environmental factors, 104, 178, 220
environmental influences, 182
environmental threats, 168
environments, 62, 104, 153, 160, 172, 185
epidemiologic, 64, 203
epidemiologic studies, 64
epigenetics, 193

Index 229

epilepsy, 43, 68
estrangement, 95, 109
ethnicity, 72, 194
etiology, 158, 159
evidence, vi, 11, 17, 48, 63, 64, 72, 135, 136, 137, 142, 146, 147, 148, 149, 151, 163, 166, 179, 184, 186, 201, 203, 204
executive function, 31, 35, 44, 60, 62, 68
exposure, 20, 29, 49, 61, 66, 79, 86, 87, 88, 92, 93, 94, 97, 101, 102, 109, 110, 111, 116, 117, 126, 142, 143, 144, 147, 148, 155, 158, 161, 163, 164, 165, 166, 171, 172, 185, 189, 201, 202, 203, 204
external locus of control, 167
externalizing behavior, 137
eye movement, 148, 152, 201
Eye Movement Desensitization and Reprocessing (EMDR), 17, 148, 149, 152, 201, 203

F

face validity, 109
families, 6, 13, 46, 141, 144, 146, 147, 151, 170, 173, 180, 182, 183, 188, 189, 193, 212
family environment, 170
family members, 160, 188
family relationships, 101
family system, 170
family therapy, 193
family violence, 20, 201, 204
fear, 8, 10, 31, 41, 93, 95, 111, 112, 114, 127, 145, 160, 168, 171, 187, 200
Federal Highway Administration, 59, 60, 75
feedback inhibition, 12
feelings, 13, 87, 95, 109, 111, 114, 123, 136, 144, 148
flashbacks, 94, 97, 109, 123, 136, 155
food, 220, 221
food security, 221
Ford, Henry, ix, xi, 4, 14, 15, 20, 68, 89, 131

G

gender differences, 16, 59, 132, 190
gene expression, 184
generalizability, 149
generalized anxiety disorder, 113
genetic disorders, 212
genetic predisposition, 10
Georgia, 3, 48, 197, 209
glucocorticoid receptor, 12
gradual exposure, 144
group therapy, 146
group treatment, 146
Group-based TF-CBT, 146
growth, 10, 21, 58, 154, 174, 200, 211
growth factor, 10, 200
guidance, 13, 173
guidelines, 17, 22, 112, 185, 194
guilt, 10, 95, 199

H

hallucinations, 112
head injury(ies), 85, 95, 200
head trauma, 8, 9, 86
healing, 124, 186, 188, 189, 194
health, vi, vii, xi, 20, 22, 37, 46, 57, 58, 66, 70, 87, 120, 127, 128, 129, 152, 158, 180, 186, 192, 193, 194, 199, 208, 209, 211, 212, 215, 218, 219, 220, 221
health care, 46, 70, 120, 127, 128, 129, 212
health care costs, 46, 70
health condition, 158
health effects, 66, 186
health status, 20, 22, 199
heart rate, 12, 137, 150
helplessness, 160
help-seeking, 170, 173, 195
high school, 17, 37, 45, 48, 54, 58, 64, 65, 70, 72, 73, 174, 183, 203
history, xi, 14, 15, 18, 19, 39, 43, 53, 101, 110, 111, 112, 158, 161, 162, 164, 202
Hong Kong, 213, 218, 220

hope, viii, x, 49, 144, 177, 185, 186, 188, 191, 194, 221
human development, 193, 209, 215, 218, 219, 220, 221
human remains, 94
Hurricane Katrina, 147, 152
hydrocortisone, 13, 201
hyperactivity, 31, 42, 44, 60, 68, 69, 158, 171
hyperarousal, 13, 113, 115, 138, 155, 165, 167, 171
hyperglycemia, 43
hypoglycemia, 43

I

ideal, 104, 147
identification, 34, 102, 107, 116, 171, 172
identity, 186, 194
illicit drug use, 67
immune function, 180
immune system, 186
Impact of Events Scale-Revised (IES-Revised), 138
impairments, 41, 69, 156
improvements, 147, 148
impulsive, 35, 63, 171
impulsivity, 44, 113
inattention, 44, 63, 64
incidence, 16, 69, 71, 132, 156
individual character, 181, 191
individual differences, 65, 178, 185
individualism, 181, 184
individuals, 13, 40, 87, 91, 99, 113, 115, 156, 157, 162, 169, 173, 179, 183, 195, 212
injuries, x, 5, 7, 8, 15, 16, 20, 25, 26, 27, 28, 44, 45, 46, 50, 51, 55, 58, 65, 69, 73, 74, 77, 78, 79, 81, 82, 83, 85, 86, 87, 92, 107, 114, 115, 116, 128, 129, 130, 132, 135, 136, 137, 148, 149, 150, 154, 159, 211
integration, 144, 145, 220
integrity, 17, 200, 203
Intellectual functioning, 166

intelligence, 166, 194, 202
intensive care unit, 14, 200
internalizing, 137, 141
interpersonal relationships, 181
intervention, vi, 18, 20, 22, 39, 69, 78, 110, 112, 116, 120, 125, 129, 131, 132, 135, 139, 140, 141, 142, 143, 144, 147, 148, 150, 151, 152, 160, 162, 171, 172, 183, 204
intoxication, 32, 37, 38, 52, 54
intrusions, 126, 155, 204
Ireland, ix, 3, 4, 5, 9, 14, 198
irritability, 8, 109, 115, 127, 155, 190
isolation, 162, 189
Israel, vi, xi, 3, 197, 209, 213, 215, 216, 218, 220, 222
issues, x, xi, 11, 13, 28, 30, 31, 32, 35, 37, 43, 44, 45, 54, 55, 56, 57, 158, 171, 199, 200, 212, 219, 220, 221

K

kill, 28, 29, 30, 31, 35

L

law enforcement, 54, 81
laws, 15, 31, 36, 40, 43, 45, 47, 49, 51, 53, 54, 56, 57, 58, 64, 66, 69, 71, 73, 74, 75, 180
learning, 13, 69, 86, 93, 156, 163, 164, 165, 167, 169, 172
learning difficulties, 13
learning environment, 164
left hemisphere, 165
legislation, 36, 47, 49, 56, 64
lifetime, 6, 91, 108, 110, 113, 117
light, 34, 61, 79, 179, 184
longitudinal study, 21, 131, 195
loss of consciousness, 9, 17, 200, 203

M

magnetic resonance, 200

Index 231

magnetic resonance imaging, 200
major depressive disorder, 8, 10, 18, 113
majority, 108, 129, 146, 177, 191, 198
maltreatment, 20, 116, 204
management, x, 12, 22, 42, 58, 111, 200, 201
marijuana, 41, 65, 66
material resources, 180
materials, 141, 143
media, 34, 35, 36, 94, 97
Medicaid, 18
medical, 18, 43, 50, 55, 59, 96, 98, 101, 109, 119, 120, 124, 125, 126, 127, 128, 129, 137, 152, 177, 180, 186, 194, 195, 202, 209, 211, 212, 213, 220
medical care, 220
medication, 13, 21, 44, 96, 98
medicine, 6, 58, 59, 207, 211, 212, 218, 219
mellitus, 43, 212, 222
membership, 207
memory, 19, 124, 171, 188
mental disorder, 7, 16, 18, 89, 93, 105, 107, 108, 110, 112, 113, 114, 116, 121, 122, 132, 136, 150, 174
mental health, vii, viii, 21, 78, 81, 87, 91, 100, 101, 104, 115, 119, 120, 124, 125, 126, 128, 129, 131, 132, 142, 147, 152, 155, 156, 158, 159, 160, 161, 162, 170, 173, 193, 194, 202
mental health professionals, 147, 155, 158, 159, 160, 161, 162, 173, 194
meta-analysis, 62, 65, 145, 150, 151, 202
metabolic syndrome, 19
methodology, 75, 199, 202
misunderstanding, 165
misuse, 78, 86
models, 82, 177, 178, 181, 184, 186
mood disorder, 165
mood swings, 111, 171
moral development, 182
morbidity, 7, 29, 42, 47, 55, 56, 57, 117
mortality, 26, 29, 38, 47, 55, 56, 57
motivation, 168, 180, 181, 182, 188
motor skills, 44, 68

Motor vehicle accidents (MVAs), 5, 7, 22, 33, 38, 43, 44, 45, 48, 49, 136, 139, 143, 148, 149
motor vehicle crashes, v, x, 3, 4, 5, 6, 9, 11, 14, 15, 21, 25, 26, 27, 28, 29, 32, 33, 38, 45, 55, 59, 60, 61, 63, 65, 68, 69, 70, 72, 74, 78, 88, 105, 119, 120, 121, 126, 131, 132, 198
multiple factors, 137
muscle relaxation, 144
musculoskeletal, 213

N

National Center for Education Statistics, 173
National Child Traumatic Stress Network, 171, 174
National Institutes of Health, 66
national security, 180
National Survey, 21, 40, 132
natural disaster, 142, 184, 201
near drowning, 14
negative consequences, 34, 41, 48
negative effects, 9, 12, 35
negative outcomes, 179
neglect, 108, 222
neurodevelopmental disorders, 44, 212
neuroscience, 184
neutral, 128, 139
New Zealand, 59, 61, 66, 70
next generation, 192, 218
night driving, 39, 49, 50, 71, 82
nightmares, 10, 17, 109, 123, 130, 132
noradrenergic system, 12
North America, 7, 58, 212

O

obesity, 220
obsessive-compulsive disorder, 123
opportunities, 162, 168, 170, 180
oppression, 180, 184
optimism, 60

P

pain, 128, 132, 169, 171, 187, 188, 199, 200
parental involvement, 154, 169, 170
parenting, 70, 144, 145, 169, 180
parents, 4, 8, 9, 12, 17, 18, 20, 26, 32, 34, 38, 40, 43, 48, 50, 54, 55, 63, 68, 71, 74, 77, 78, 98, 100, 101, 107, 109, 111, 117, 130, 131, 140, 141, 142, 145, 147, 150, 151, 156, 157, 162, 163, 169, 170, 172, 175, 179, 191, 194, 198, 200, 220
participants, 108, 114, 115, 140, 141, 143, 145, 146, 147
pathology, 186
pathophysiology, 200
pathways, 182, 184, 193
pedal, 77, 79, 81, 84, 85, 89
pediatrician, 87, 221
peer influence, 61, 62
peer relationship, 101, 169
Peritraumatic distress, 160
personality characteristics, 61
personality disorder, 112, 123
personality factors, 31
personality traits, 36, 63
phobia, 112, 113
physical aggression, 95, 98
physical environment, 180
physical health, 180
physical injury, 8, 12, 17, 77, 92, 110, 117, 131, 136, 157, 159, 160, 162, 175, 191, 199, 201
physicians, 86, 87, 115
pilot study, 152
PKU, 217
plaque, x, 5
plasticity, 162
playing, 29, 137, 183, 194
PM, 32, 63, 65, 66
police, 27, 38, 42, 43, 45, 54, 56, 74, 79, 80, 92, 94, 172, 180
policy, 17, 53, 83, 194, 218
poor performance, 166

population, x, 4, 9, 14, 27, 55, 79, 81, 82, 83, 86, 87, 88, 99, 110, 117, 126, 193, 194, 195, 198, 203
positive correlation, 200
positive emotions, 95, 136
positive relationship, 159
posttraumatic play, 109
posttraumatic stress, v, vi, 7, 12, 14, 17, 18, 19, 20, 21, 91, 94, 97, 99, 105, 116, 117, 120, 121, 124, 125, 126, 128, 129, 131, 132, 135, 136, 137, 138, 141, 142, 148, 150, 151, 152, 156, 157, 174, 175, 195, 202
posttraumatic stress disorder (PTSD), v, vi, x, 6, 7, 8, 9, 10, 11, 12, 13, 14, 17, 18, 19, 20, 21, 22, 54, 91, 92, 93, 94, 99, 100, 101, 102, 103, 104, 105, 107, 108, 109, 110, 111, 112, 113, 114, 115, 116, 117, 119, 120, 121, 122, 123, 124, 125, 126, 127, 128, 129, 130, 131, 132, 135, 136,137, 138, 139, 140, 141, 142, 143, 144, 145, 146, 147, 148, 149, 150, 151, 152, 155, 156, 157, 158, 159, 160, 161, 162, 163, 166, 167, 169, 170, 171, 174, 175, 177, 178, 185, 187, 189, 195, 198, 202, 203, 204190, 191, 195, 198, 199, 200, 201, 202, 203, 204
posttraumatic stress symptoms, 17, 19, 20, 105, 124, 125, 129, 132, 137, 141, 150, 156, 174
poverty, 182
predictability, 170, 171
preschool, 18, 21, 102, 107, 109, 116, 132, 141, 150, 151, 203
preschool children, 18, 21, 107, 109, 132, 151, 203
prescription drugs, 51
prevalence, 13, 25, 37, 40, 41, 51, 52, 61, 64, 66, 69, 73, 91, 101, 105, 110, 114, 115, 119, 120, 122, 130, 155, 156, 157, 161, 169, 190, 198, 199
prevalence rate, 130, 157
prevention, vii, 13, 34, 42, 57, 61, 63, 64, 65, 70, 71, 73, 89, 136, 143, 145, 173, 192, 194, 201, 209, 221

primary caregivers, 97, 153, 154
principles, x, 42, 56
problem-solving, 141, 144, 171, 180, 190
procedural justice, 73
professionals, 116, 131, 177, 186, 216, 218
protection, 55, 180, 192, 195, 211
protective factors, 39, 110, 179, 181, 182, 190, 191
psychiatric comorbidity, 107, 108, 113, 117, 203
psychiatric disorders, 199, 201
psychiatric morbidity, 7
psychiatry, 174
psychoactive drug, 38
psychological development, 60
psychological distress, 18, 93, 94, 97, 99, 174, 190, 202
Psychological impact, 126
psychological problems, 6, 8, 10, 108, 125, 181
psychological stress, 77, 79, 80, 86, 87, 88, 93
psychologist, vii, 119, 173, 208
psychology, 178
psychopathology, 10, 13, 17, 19, 69, 132, 140, 141, 142, 148, 150, 175, 179, 192, 193, 199, 202
psychopharmacology, 13, 212, 222
psychosocial development, 108
psychosocial dysfunction, 147
psychotropic medications, 35
PTSD, v, vi, x, 6, 7, 8, 9, 10, 11, 12, 13, 14, 17, 18, 19, 20, 21, 22, 54, 91, 92, 93, 94, 99, 100, 101, 102, 103, 104, 105, 107, 108, 109, 110, 111, 112, 113, 114, 115, 116, 117, 119, 120, 121, 122, 123, 124, 125, 126, 127, 128, 129, 130, 131, 132, 135, 136,137, 138, 139, 140, 141, 142, 143, 144, 145, 146, 147, 148, 149, 150, 151, 152, 155, 156, 157, 158, 159, 160, 161, 162, 163, 166, 167, 169, 170, 171, 174, 175, 177, 178, 185, 187, 189, 190, 191, 195, 198, 199, 200, 201, 202, 203, 204
PTSD subtype, 107

public health, 37, 59, 180, 184, 209, 215, 216, 218, 219, 220, 221
public schools, 173
public service, 215
punishment, 42, 53, 54, 125, 126

Q

qualifications, 93
quality of life, 12, 13, 20, 22, 199, 209
query, 173
questionnaire, 9

R

race, 34, 72, 193, 194
random assignment, 183
reactions, 12, 13, 16, 17, 87, 94, 97, 111, 115, 121, 122, 127, 128, 131, 132, 136, 139, 140, 141, 142, 147, 157, 174
reactivity, 95, 98, 127, 136, 137, 191
reality, 158, 201
recidivism, 53, 73
recognition, 6, 7, 12, 144, 207
recommendations, 107, 159
reconstruction, 139, 141
recovery, 20, 130, 141, 154, 157, 160, 162, 163, 186, 188, 193, 195, 202
recovery process, 154, 163, 189
recreational, 180, 182
reenactment, 94, 97, 109, 121, 122, 124
rehabilitation, 209, 215
relaxation, 143, 144, 146, 147, 149
reprocessing, 152, 201
requirements, 45, 72, 104
researchers, 4, 7, 12, 14, 29, 42, 44, 143, 181, 182, 183, 184, 198, 199, 219
resilience, x, 48, 70, 110, 147, 177, 178, 179, 180, 181, 182, 183, 184, 185, 186, 188, 191, 192, 193, 194, 195
resources, 57, 78, 81, 83, 100, 101, 147, 149, 162, 164, 179, 181, 184, 185, 186, 188, 212

response, 32, 80, 93, 95, 98, 99, 102, 103, 104, 112, 116, 124, 126, 127, 129, 130, 137, 150, 156, 163, 164, 165, 166, 167, 168, 172, 178, 186, 187, 189, 190
restrictions, 36, 49, 50, 71, 101
restructuring, 143
right hemisphere, 165
risk, 5, 6, 8, 9, 12, 13, 18, 25, 26, 30, 31, 32, 33, 36, 38, 39, 41, 42, 43, 44, 46, 47, 48, 51, 58, 59, 60, 61, 62, 63, 64, 65, 66, 68, 69, 70, 71, 72, 73, 74, 75, 83, 84, 85, 113, 117, 122, 123, 125, 128, 132, 135, 137, 138, 139, 142, 145, 148, 149, 150, 153, 156, 159, 160, 161, 162, 163, 178, 179, 181, 182, 185, 190, 191, 192, 194, 200, 203, 204
risk assessment, 161
risk factors, 18, 32, 36, 66, 68, 110, 116, 117, 137, 150, 156, 162, 179, 182, 183, 185, 194, 195, 204
risk perception, 59, 60, 61, 63
risk taking, 6, 32, 44, 59, 60, 61
risk-taking, 30, 60
routines, 170, 171, 189

S

safety, ix, x, 5, 9, 15, 17, 31, 34, 44, 46, 47, 49, 55, 56, 58, 59, 60, 68, 69, 70, 71, 74, 75, 77, 78, 82, 88, 89, 104, 144, 145, 147, 160, 161, 167, 168, 169, 171, 172, 191
scholarship, 182, 207
school, 8, 17, 37, 40, 43, 45, 48, 50, 56, 68, 86, 98, 101, 104, 108, 109, 110, 113, 117, 125, 127, 137, 145, 147, 152, 153, 154, 155, 156, 157, 159, 160, 161, 162, 163, 164, 165, 166, 167, 168, 169, 170, 172, 173, 174, 181, 182, 185, 189, 193, 198, 200, 218, 219, 220
school adjustment, 101
school performance, 108, 170
science, 184, 192, 216
screen for PTSD, 115
seat belt use, 39, 45, 54, 56, 69

security, 172
seeking safety, 56
self-assessment, 103
self-control, 31
self-destructive behavior, 95, 137
self-efficacy, 128, 133, 144
self-esteem, 183, 186
self-organization, 192
self-regulation, 31, 180
sensing, 109, 167
sensitivity, 34, 41, 111, 200, 204
services, 101, 115, 146, 159, 160, 170, 180, 184, 194
sexual experiences, 122
sexual health, 212
sexual violence, 94, 97, 127, 136
sexuality, 221
signs, 64, 69, 86, 87, 107, 109, 112, 120, 153, 159, 160, 163, 170, 172
skull fracture, 16
sleep apnea, 43, 68
sleep deprivation, 35
sleep disorders, 43, 68
sleep disturbance, 137
sleep latency, 130
social context, 17, 182
social control, 126
social environment, 60
social norms, 14, 22, 49
social relationships, 167
social services, 180
social skills, 144
social support, 119, 121, 125, 162, 163, 169, 170, 178, 182, 190, 191, 194
social support network, 190
social withdrawal, 109, 126, 171
socialization, 178
society, x, 4, 6, 9, 14, 26, 38, 41, 42, 43, 55, 57, 198, 201, 216
socioeconomic status, 137, 181
Somatic complaints, 171
specialists, 211
specifications, 93, 102
speculation, 41
spending, 168

stability, 46, 55, 122, 170, 180
stabilization, 144
states, 35, 38, 39, 40, 43, 49, 50, 51, 53, 55, 56, 64, 67, 68, 71, 72, 122, 165, 173
statistics, x, 26, 55, 78, 79, 80, 81, 83, 85, 87, 88, 92, 110, 173
stepped-care TF-CBT (SC-TF-CBT), 146
stigma, 189
stimulation, 148
stimulus discrimination, 143
strength-based, 177, 186, 187, 188, 191
stress, v, vi, x, xi, 6, 7, 8, 9, 10, 11, 12, 13, 14, 15, 16, 17, 18, 19, 20, 21, 22, 42, 54, 57, 91, 92, 93, 94, 99, 100, 101, 102, 103, 104, 105, 107, 108, 109, 110, 111, 112, 113, 114, 115, 116, 117, 119, 120, 121, 122, 123, 124, 125, 126, 127, 128, 129, 130,131, 132, 135, 136, 137, 138, 139, 140, 141, 142, 143, 144, 145, 146, 147, 148, 149, 150, 151, 152, 155, 156, 157, 158, 159, 160, 161, 162, 163, 166, 167, 169, 170, 171, 174, 175, 177, 178, 180, 182, 184, 185, 187, 188, 189, 190, 191, 193, 195, 198, 199, 200, 201, 202, 203, 204
stress reactions, 16, 113, 117, 120, 132, 140, 141, 204
stress response, 18, 19, 110, 112, 180
stressors, 162, 185
structure, 10, 12, 105, 110, 143, 171, 180, 200
styles, 10, 21, 46, 48, 71, 167, 175
subgroups, 31, 200
subjective experience, 187
substance abuse, 111, 116
Substance Abuse and Mental Health Services Administration (SAMHSA), 40
substance use, 42, 65, 73, 183
suicidal ideation, 113
suicide, vii, 5, 14, 26, 123, 188, 195, 221
supervision, 33, 50, 51, 169
suppression, 124, 126
surveillance, 88
survival rate, 186
survivors, vi, 6, 15, 21, 117, 150, 153, 154, 155, 156, 157, 158, 159, 160, 162, 166, 168, 169, 170, 172, 173, 174, 175, 186, 203
susceptibility, 17, 161
sustainability, 168
symptoms, 7, 8, 11, 12, 13, 17, 18, 19, 20, 21, 79, 87, 91, 93, 94, 97, 100, 101, 102, 103, 104, 105, 107, 109, 110, 111, 112, 113, 114, 115, 116, 120, 122, 123, 124, 125, 127, 128, 129, 130, 131, 132, 136, 137, 138, 139, 140, 141, 142, 143, 144, 145, 146, 147, 148, 149, 150, 152, 153, 155, 156, 157, 158, 159, 160, 161, 162, 163, 164, 165, 169, 170, 171, 172, 174, 175, 177, 178, 185, 186, 188, 189, 190, 191, 195, 200, 202, 203
syndrome, 9, 12, 192, 204

T

tactile stimuli, 148
teachers, x, 130, 147, 153, 155, 156, 159, 161, 164, 165, 166, 170, 172, 173, 182, 194, 200
teacher-student relationship, 164
technology, 30, 35, 36, 44, 46, 47, 48, 55, 56, 63, 82
teens, 31, 32, 33, 45, 61, 63, 65, 68, 69, 74, 80, 83
temperament, 180
temporal lobe, 12
terrorism, 184, 192
text messaging, 34, 63
therapeutic effect, 125
therapeutic relationship, 144
therapist, 144, 146
therapy, vii, 13, 17, 36, 140, 142, 143, 144, 145, 146, 147, 149, 151, 152, 201, 203
thoughts, 95, 111, 113, 123, 125, 127, 136, 137, 139, 144, 148, 166, 167
threats, 145, 161, 168, 172, 182
training, 33, 34, 42, 47, 48, 49, 50, 51, 61, 70, 83, 115, 130, 143, 145, 147, 149, 172, 186, 208, 216

training programs, 48, 61
traits, 44, 182, 183
transformation, 211
transportation, 6, 14, 29, 42, 52, 154, 167, 168, 171
trauma, x, 4, 7, 8, 9, 10, 11, 12, 13, 14, 16, 17, 18, 19, 20, 21, 77, 79, 80, 83, 86, 87, 91, 92, 93, 94, 97, 99, 100, 101, 103, 105, 108, 109, 110, 111, 112, 115, 116, 119, 120, 121, 122, 123, 124, 125, 126, 127, 128, 129, 130, 131, 132, 133, 136, 137, 139, 140, 141, 142, 143, 144, 145, 146, 147, 148, 149, 150, 151, 152, 153, 155, 156, 157, 158, 159, 160, 161, 162, 163, 164, 165, 166, 167, 169, 170, 171, 172, 173, 174, 179, 185, 187, 188, 189, 190, 194, 195, 198, 199, 200, 201, 202, 203, 204
trauma history, 111, 161, 162, 164
trauma narrative, 144, 145, 147
Trauma-focused cognitive behavioral therapy (TF-CBT), 142, 143, 144, 145, 146, 147
traumatic brain injury (TBI), 9, 17, 42, 43, 44, 132, 135, 136, 200, 203
traumatic events, 13, 94, 97, 102, 108, 110, 111, 112, 113, 116, 120, 128, 136, 139, 145, 151, 153, 158, 161, 178, 189
traumatic experiences, 103, 162, 198, 200
traumatic incident, 102
treatment, vii, viii, 7, 11, 12, 13, 17, 20, 42, 88, 92, 100, 104, 111, 112, 116, 120, 121, 135, 136, 137, 140, 141, 142, 143, 144, 145, 146, 147, 148, 149, 150, 159, 170, 195, 200, 201, 203, 204, 208
trial, 20, 60, 72, 131, 132, 140, 150, 151, 152
triggers, 136, 144, 145, 172
truck drivers, 44, 69
type 1 diabetes, 43, 68

U

U.S. Centers for Disease Control and Prevention, 40

underlying mechanisms, 194
unintentional injuries, 5, 26, 27, 57, 75, 136
United States (USA), vi, viii, ix, xi, 3, 4, 5, 6, 7, 14, 15, 25, 26, 27, 28, 29, 33, 35, 37, 39, 40, 44, 47, 51, 57, 58, 59, 61, 62, 63, 64, 65, 68, 69, 71, 72, 74, 77, 78, 80, 91, 107, 108, 110, 115, 117, 119, 120, 135, 136, 149, 153, 154, 173, 177, 178, 181, 197, 198, 201, 207, 208, 209, 211, 213, 217
urban, 28, 34, 41, 48, 62, 83, 84
US Department of Health and Human Services, 116

V

variables, 20, 189, 199
vehicles, ix, x, 4, 5, 6, 9, 16, 26, 27, 28, 29, 31, 34, 36, 44, 46, 47, 55, 56, 57, 62, 69, 74, 77, 80, 81, 83, 85, 127, 135, 154, 198, 202
Verbal skills, 165
victimization, 108, 173
victims, 8, 13, 16, 17, 20, 42, 58, 114, 115, 117, 149, 174, 199, 203, 204
violence, 13, 14, 22, 29, 108, 122, 143, 147, 152, 174, 180, 201, 220
violent behavior, 190
visual acuity, 60
vulnerability, 110, 193

W

walking, 83, 84
war, 36, 88, 129, 192
Washington, 16, 59, 60, 65, 66, 116, 132, 150, 174, 191
wear, 44, 46, 57
web, 88, 141, 149, 151
web-based intervention, 141
Wechsler Intelligence Scale, 166
welfare, 81, 180, 209, 215
well-being, 194, 209, 222
white matter, 9, 17, 200, 203

working memory, 44
World Health Organization, 81
worry, 11, 126, 169, 171

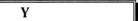

young adults, 29, 35, 37, 38, 41, 60, 69, 105, 154, 212
young people, 39, 151, 177, 181, 191, 220